EXPANDING WAISTLINES

TRANSGRESSIONS: CULTURAL STUDIES AND EDUCATION
Volume 17

Scope

Cultural studies provides an analytical toolbox for both making sense of educational practice and extending the insights of educational professionals into their labors. In this context *Transgressions: Cultural Studies and Education* provides a collection of books in the domain that specify this assertion. Crafted for an audience of teachers, teacher educators, scholars and students of cultural studies and others interested in cultural studies and pedagogy, the series documents both the possibilities of and the controversies surrounding the intersection of cultural studies and education. The editors and the authors of this series do not assume that the interaction of cultural studies and education devalues other types of knowledge and analytical forms. Rather the intersection of these knowledge disciplines offers a rejuvenating, optimistic, and positive perspective on education and educational institutions. Some might describe its contribution as democratic, emancipatory, and transformative. The editors and authors maintain that cultural studies helps free educators from sterile, monolithic analyses that have for too long undermined efforts to think of educational practices by providing other words, new languages, and fresh metaphors. Operating in an interdisciplinary cosmos, Transgressions: Cultural Studies and Education is dedicated to exploring the ways cultural studies enhances the study and practice of education. With this in mind the series focuses in a non-exclusive way on popular culture as well as other dimensions of cultural studies including social theory, social justice and positionality, cultural dimensions of technological innovation, new media and media literacy, new forms of oppression emerging in an electronic hyperreality, and postcolonial global concerns. With these concerns in mind cultural studies scholars often argue that the realm of popular culture is the most powerful educational force in contemporary culture. Indeed, in the twenty-first century this pedagogical dynamic is sweeping through the entire world. Educators, they believe, must understand these emerging realities in order to gain an important voice in the pedagogical conversation.

Without an understanding of cultural pedagogy's (education that takes place outside of formal schooling) role in the shaping of individual identity--youth identity in particular--the role educators play in the lives of their students will continue to fade. Why do so many of our students feel that life is incomprehensible and devoid of meaning? What does it mean, teachers wonder, when young people are unable to describe their moods, their affective affiliation to the society around them. Meanings provided young people by mainstream institutions often do little to help them deal with their affective complexity, their difficulty negotiating the rift between meaning and affect. School knowledge and educational expectations seem as anachronistic as a ditto machine, not that learning ways of rational thought and making sense of the world are unimportant.

But school knowledge and educational expectations often have little to offer students about making sense of the way they feel, the way their affective lives are shaped. In no way do we argue that analysis of the production of youth in an electronic mediated world demands some "touchy-feely" educational superficiality. What is needed in this context is a rigorous analysis of the interrelationship between pedagogy, popular culture, meaning making, and youth subjectivity. In an era marked by youth depression, violence, and suicide such insights become extremely important, even life saving. Pessimism about the future is the common sense of many contemporary youth with its concomitant feeling that no one can make a difference.

If affective production can be shaped to reflect these perspectives, then it can be reshaped to lay the groundwork for optimism, passionate commitment, and transformative educational and political activity. In these ways cultural studies adds a dimension to the work of education unfilled by any other sub-discipline. This is what Transgressions: Cultural Studies and Education seeks to produce— literature on these issues that makes a difference. It seeks to publish studies that help those who work with young people, those individuals involved in the disciplines that study children and youth, and young people themselves improve their lives in these bizarre times.

Volume 1
An Unordinary Death...*The Life of a Suicide Bomber*
Khalilah Christina Sabra
Paperback ISBN 90-77874-36-4 Hardback ISBN 90-77874-37-2

Volume 2
Lyrical Minded
The Critical Pedagogy of Hip-Hop Artist KRS-ONE
Priya Parmar, City University of New York, USA
Paperback ISBN 90-77874-50-X Hardback ISBN 90-77874-64-X

Volume 3
Pedagogy and Praxis in the Age of Empire
Towards a New Humanism
Peter McLaren & Nathalia Jaramillo
Paperback ISBN 90-77874-84-4 Hardback ISBN 90-77874-85-2

Expanding Waistlines

An Educator's Guide to Childhood Obesity

By

David Campos
University of the Incarnate Word

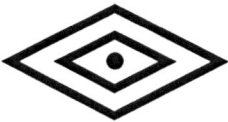

SENSE PUBLISHERS
ROTTERDAM / TAIPEI

A C.I.P. record for this book is available from the Library of Congress.

ISBN 978-90-8790-206-3 (paperback)
ISBN 978-90-8790-207-0 (hardback)
ISBN 978-90-8790-208-7 (e-book)

Published by: Sense Publishers,
P.O. Box 21858, 3001 AW Rotterdam, The Netherlands
http://www.sensepublishers.com

Printed on acid-free paper

To my mother, Guadalupe, who gives me strength, confidence, and a sense of social responsibility

TABLE OF CONTENTS

PART III. RESOURCES

PREFACE AND ACKNOWLEDGEMENTS

PREFACE

I accepted a job in San Antonio and moved from Chicago in August 2003. I had been a classroom teacher in the early nineties and continued to work with children and teachers as an associate professor of education. When I began the academic year that fall I entered many classrooms like I had for over a dozen years supervising student teachers and teaching field-based courses. But this particular time I made an observation that left me worried: many of the children in the classrooms were overweight and some were obese. My observations were not isolated to one classroom, one school, or one district. Overweight children were seemingly everywhere.

When I was a second grade teacher, there may have been a child per grade level who was heavyset and I was not concerned one bit. After all, I know that there are thin, tall, and short people, and some who happen to be overweight. The same holds true for children, so I thought. But this time, I could not reconcile what I remembered from my teaching days to the apparent pattern that I was noticing before my very eyes. I purposely decided to investigate childhood obesity when I saw two disturbing incidents. The first occurred when I was dining at a popular Tex-Mex restaurant and I saw a very large four-year girl eating from her own adult plate with adult-sized portions. I later noted that she was eating a tamale wrapped in a tortilla and drinking a strawberry-cream soda. The girl was cute as can be, and her family was evidently smitten with her. But, adjectives like plump, chubby, or big-boned could not mask that she was obese.

Within a week or two, I was dining at a popular buffet-style diner known for their fresh salads, soups, and quasi-healthy desserts. While there I saw a very large 12-year-old boy eating with his mother. My initial thought was, "Aha, now there's a mother who is conscientious about her son's health and wants to do something to promote a well-balanced diet!" At the heels of that thought, I noticed that he had not chosen the wonderful greens or the wholesome soups, but was eating Italian bread sticks that he dunked into a bowl of Alfredo sauce. As far as I could tell he had eaten nearly a dozen before he made his own dessert: a mound of cubed pound cakes poured over with chocolate syrup (both were intended for the non-fat frozen yogurt). Somehow, like a warrior who skillfully avoids mines in a field, the boy had deflected all the healthy vegetables, fruit, and side dishes. The boy—much like his counterpart at the Tex-Mex restaurant—was unmistakably obese.

My heart went out to these two and children like them because I thought about their self-esteem, their self-confidence, their physical limitations, and how they might feel when they compare themselves to others. Not to mention, the emotional turmoil they must deal with when others tease or insult them like children often do. I had not even considered the medical risks they face when they have excess weight. I began to read up on childhood obesity and ask my teacher friends whether they perceive obesity or overweight a problem in their schools. Unsurprisingly, they had noticed that children were seemingly heavier, but in the world of high-stakes testing and all the other instructional and extra-curricular demands they encounter, many of them had not considered childhood obesity a critical dilemma. One teacher made an interesting point, "You begin to accept the heavier weight as normal so that it doesn't even cross your mind that we should do something about it. Plus, the role models in their lives –parents, family members, teachers, members in their community, etc.—are overweight too. So, it becomes perfectly acceptable to be fat and grow up fat when everyone around you is fat. So, why rush to curb childhood obesity when it's pervasive among adults?" The answer is simple. Children with healthy weight will have a better quality of life.

All of these circumstances led me to write this book to inform teachers and other youth-advocates about childhood obesity. I wanted school personnel to have this primer on the topic so that they could fully understand childhood obesity and have the background knowledge to guide children and adolescents toward a healthy lifestyle. I divided *Expanding Waistlines* into three sections. Part I, the overview, is comprised of three chapters that give background information on the childhood obesity crisis. Readers can learn about the topic and make their way toward the associated risks and predictors. Part II, health promotion, encompasses three chapters devoted to promoting health at school and home. Part III, is the resource chapter, which outlines print and online resources and health advocacy organizations. I have learned a great deal about childhood obesity; I hope readers will do the same.

ACKNOWLEDGEMENTS

I could not have written this book without the generous support from a number of people. I am indebted to my father and mother, Agapito and Guadalupe, for their unconditional love. Throughout my life they have made it easy for me to accomplish what I need and like to do. Likewise, I remain grateful to my brothers Ernie and John for their unwavering encouragement and tireless support. I am very fortunate to have such a caring family that embraces me with warmth, compassion, respect, and love. I also appreciate my friends Simon Chow, Alex Clemenzi, Bobby Coronado, Koran Kanaifu, and Ericka Knudson who always bring much-needed balance in my life.

I would also like to thank my colleague and friend Dr. Valerie Janesick who inspires me and deepens my understanding of scholarship. I am appreciative of my friend Dr. Ken A. Perez for his constructive comments on early drafts of the manuscript. His suggestions and insight from the physician's perspective were consistently on target. I extend a special thanks to my graduate assistant Elizabeth Clemons for her help in gathering materials and her contribution to Chapter 3, the genetics tutorial (Table 9). She is an amazingly positive and enthusiastic teacher. I also offer my sincerest appreciation to my editor Joe Kincheloe for his expert guidance and seeing this through to production. Lastly, I wish to thank to my vice president of academic affairs, Dr. Denise Doyle, who funded my graduate assistant and a course release that ultimately afforded me time to finish this book.

CHAPTER 1

INTRODUCTION

A TROUBLING TREND

One of the biggest health concerns of our time impacts the lives of youth. A growing number of youth are out of shape and the girth of their waists is becoming wider. With as many as six million American youth considered overweight to the point that their health is endangered and another five million who are at risk of becoming overweight, there are no signs of the increasing trend slowing down. Childhood obesity has become a serious matter that is becoming widespread, and if left unchallenged will produce an unprecedented generation that has dire medical problems, including psychosocial concerns associated with weight gain.

Since the 1970s, obesity prevalence has more than doubled for youth in the 2 to 5 year-old and the 12 to 19 year-old classes, and more than tripled for youth who are 6 to 11 years old. Experts believe that varying factors contribute to this complex epidemic ranging from excessive consumption of high calorie, refined foods to limited physical activity. Concerned with the poor choices that some overweight youth make, a number of federal, state, and professional organizations are engaged in prevention and intervention initiatives to help transform children's eating habits and exercise behaviors. While transforming behaviors is never easy, long-term aggressive attempts to reduce the obesity rates are certainly worthwhile if we expect future generations to be healthy and active.

This introductory chapter explores childhood obesity by addressing the following:
- What is childhood obesity and why should I be concerned?
- Why is childhood obesity on the rise?
- How is childhood obesity measured?
- What is being done to combat childhood obesity?

WHAT IS CHILHDOOD OBESITY AND WHY SHOULD I BE CONCERNED?

Childhood obesity has received considerable publicity in the last decade for good reason. The prevalence of overweight and obese children has skyrocketed driving many health officials, including the World Health Organization, to term this critical problem an epidemic (Wake, Hesketh & Waters, 2003). In fact, childhood obesity is emerging as one of the most alarming public health concerns of our time. The United States Surgeon General (US Department of Health & Human Services, 2005c), the American Academy of Pediatrics (2003), the Food and Nutrition and Consumer Services Undersecretary of the USDA (Crane, 2004), and a host of other health authorities recognize that childhood obesity is unprecedented in our history and if left unresolved will become a giant burden on American health.

But when exactly is a child considered obese? The public health community uses various definitions to describe the population that is heavier than average. There is no clearly established, accepted or agreed upon definition of childhood obesity (Broadwater, 2002; Goodman, Hinden, & Khandelwal, 2000; Mast et al, 2002). In simple terms, however, childhood obesity is the state of being overweight due to excess body weight – presumably excess muscles, bone, fat, and water – in proportion to a person's height (Montague, 2003). Some have noted that children who are heavier than 120 percent of the average weight for a particular height, gender, and age are obese (Jalongo, 1999). Others, such as the Center for Disease Control and Prevention (CDC) avoid the term *obese* and instead use *overweight* when referring to children because of its negative connotation.

The CDC and the World Health Organization, the American Heart Association, and others use the body mass index (BMI) formula to measure obesity. The BMI, which is calculated as the weight (in kilograms) divided by the height (in meters, squared), has become the most commonly used tool to distinguish overweight and obese children. In fact, BMI reference charts, which factor age and growth patterns, have been published for children in Germany, North America, France, the United Kingdom, Sweden, and Italy. While these charts are widely used, there is no uniform demarcation between overweight and obesity. For instance:

- The Centers for Disease Control and Prevention classifies children who are "at risk of being overweight" if their BMI is above the 95th percentile for their sex and age, and "overweight" if their BMI is between the 85th and 95th percentile;
- The American Heart Association distinguishes children whose BMI is equal to or greater than the 85th percentile as mildly to moderately overweight, those whose BMI falls between the 85th and 95th percentiles as at risk for obesity, and those whose BMI is equal to or greater than the 95th percentile are considered obese;
- The American Obesity Association (2005) writes, "The AOA uses the 95th percentile as criteria for obesity because it corresponds to a BMI of 30 which is obesity in adults. The 85th percentile corresponds to a BMI of 25, adult overweight"
- According to Mast et al. (2002), some medical professionals use the 90th BMI percentile for overweight, 97.5[th] percentile for obesity, and 75th for screening "preobese" children.

The latest statistical data underscore that childhood obesity is not unique to the United States – it is a widespread issue throughout the developed and developing world (Hardus, Van Vuuren, Crawford, & Worsley, 2003). In Australia, for example, the prevalence of overweight children has doubled and childhood obesity has tripled from 1985 to 1995, with roughly a quarter of Australian children (2 and 17 years old) considered overweight or obese (Hardus, et al.). In Canada, the number of overweight children (a BMI greater than the 85th percentile) more than doubled from 1981 to 1996 with the prevalence of overweight boys increasing from 15% to 28.8%, and 15% to 23.8% for girls. During this time, the prevalence of obese children more than doubled from 5% to 13.55% for boys and 11.8% for girls (Gillis, Kennedy, Gillis, & Bar-Or, 2002). The number of Japanese obese children (6 to 14 years old) has also increased from 5% to 10% between 1974 and 1993 (Deckelbaum & Williams, 2001), and in Taiwan the prevalence of obesity for boys and girls between 9 and 11 years old was about 17.9% and 17.7% respectively (Wu, Yu, Wei, & Yin, 2003). Surprisingly, even Ireland, Greece, Portugal and countries in North Africa, Eastern Asia, and South America find a rising trend in obesity. After analyzing worldwide trends, the International Obesity Task Force predicts that about 38% of all European children will be overweight by the year 2010 (Egan, 2007). There are about 22 million children under 5 years-old who are overweight worldwide (Deckelbaum & Williams).

The number of overweight and obese children in the United States is staggering. Current estimates suggest that roughly 22 percent of American youth (6- to 19-years old) are overweight, which is about nine million youth or one youth in five (U.S. Department of Health & Human Services, 2005; Institute of Medicine, 2005). In the 2- to 5 year-old class, about 10% are considered overweight (Kaiser Family Foundation, 2004). The rates of childhood obesity have increased dramatically over the past four decades, in some instances double and triple the proportions of those reported in 1960s and 1970s. Between 1963-1965, for instance, about 5% of youth between 12- and 19-year olds were considered obese (Lederman, Akabas, & Moore, 2004). But between 1988 and 1994, the prevalence increased to 11%, and to 15.5% by 1999-2000. Table 1 presents the Centers for Disease Control data from the National Health and Nutrition Examination Surveys (I, II, III), which report (in cycles) the proportion of children who are overweight. Contrasted with the figures in Table 2, the National Center for Health Statistics data, it becomes evident that childhood obesity is increasingly prevalent.

Table 1. Prevalence of overweight and obese children[i]

Cycle Year	Prevalence of Children Who Are Overweight (>= 85th Percentile of BMI)		Prevalence of Children Who Are Obese (>=95th Percentile of BMI)	
	6-11 year olds	12-17 year olds	6-11 year olds	12-17 year olds
1963-1965	15	15	5	5
1966-1970	15	15	5	5
1988-1991	22	22	11	11.5

Table 2. Percentages of childhood obesity[ii]

	Percent of Obese 6-11 Year-olds	*Percent of Obese 12-19 Year-olds*
1963-1970	4	5
1971-1974	4	6
1976-1980	7	5
1988-1994	11	11
1999-2000	15	15

This phenomenon is not unique to children; obesity has increased dramatically among adults too. Rates of adult obesity rose from 25% in the 1970s to 33% in the 1980s (Gable & Lutz, 2000). Data from NHANES 1999-2000 find that an estimated 60 million adults over the age of 20 were obese because their BMI was 30 or greater (National Center for Health Statistics, 2004), and other data indicated that about 61% of adults had a BMI greater than 25 leaving them classified as overweight or obese (U.S. Department of Health & Human Service, 2005a). In all, roughly 97 million adults in the U.S. are overweight (Davis, Davis, Northington, Moll, & Kolar, 2002) with the average American adult gaining about two pounds each year (Peters, Wyatt, Donahoo, & Hill, 2002). Table 3 ranks the states by the percent of obese residents from least to greatest.

Health authorities are alarmed for good reason. Children and adolescents who are overweight or obese are at risk for a host of adverse health problems. Experts agree that obesity represents a chronic disease and fear that this population of overweight children will live shorter, more diseased lives than generations before (Cafazzo, 2005). In fact, the federal government has isolated obesity as the second leading cause of illness and premature death rivaling smoking and use of tobacco products. Currently, as many as one out of eight deaths in America, or roughly 325,000 people, is caused from an illness directly related to being overweight or obese (U.S. Department of Health & Human Services, 2003; Maddock, 2004).

The American Academy of Pediatrics (2003) explain that obesity is a burden on children's health because those who are excessively heavy risk complex, multifaceted health problems. Some of the medical complications common among overweight children include adverse effects on growth, blood pressure, blood lipids, cholesterol, and glucose metabolism leading to a greater risk of hypertension, hyperlipidemis, type 2 diabetes, and cardiovascular diseases. Other ailments include respiratory problems such as asthma and obstructive sleep apnea, bone and joint problems (especially in the lower body), gall bladder diseases, stroke, certain types of cancer, gout, and other chronic conditions (Kaiser Family Foundation, 2004; Thorpe, List, Marx, May, Helgerson, & Frieden, 2004).

Being overweight also affects the human spirit because extra pounds and a larger size are a stigma in our society. Many persons, including children, associate being overweight with being lazy, having little self-control, incompetence, and incapable of moving with ease. Today, in playgrounds across the nation, children will use epithets like "fatso," "hippo," and "fatty" to degrade one another. It should

Table 3. State rankings by percentages of obese residents and youth[iii]

State Rank	% of Obese Residents	State Rank	% of Overweight or Obese 10- to 17-Year-olds
1. Colorado	16.5	1. Utah	21
2. Hawaii	17.1	2. Colorado	22
3. Utah	17.5	3. Wyoming	23
4. New Hampshire	17.9	4. Minnesota	24
5. Connecticut	18.0	5. Washington	25
6. Massachusetts	18.3	6. South Dakota	26
7. Rhode Island	18.5	6. Idaho	26
8. Montana	18.7	6. Vermont	26
9. Vermont	18.9	6. Iowa	26
10. New Jersey	19.0	6. Oregon	26
11. California	19.2	6. Nebraska	26
12. Florida	19.4	12. Nevada	27
13. Maryland	19.4	12. Connecticut	27
14. Wyoming	19.5	12. Rhode Island	27
15. Arizona	19.6	12. New Hampshire	27
16. New Mexico	19.7	12. Hawaii	27
17. Idaho	20.2	12. North Dakota	27
18. Oregon	20.3	12. Montana	27
19. New York	20.6	19. Oklahoma	28
20. Delaware	20.7	20. Pennsylvania	29
21. Maine	20.7	20. Wisconsin	29
22. South Dakota	21.2	20. New Mexico	29
23. Washington	21.3	20. Massachusetts	29
24. Nevada	21.6	20. Michigan	29
25. Wisconsin	21.6	25. Maine	30
26. Illinois	21.9	25. Maryland	30
27. District of Columbia	22.4	25. Arizona	30
28. Minnesota	22.4	25. Ohio	30
29. Kansas	22.8	25. Virginia	30
30. Iowa	22.9	25. California	30
31. Oklahoma	22.9	25. Kansas	30
32. Ohio	23.0	32. New York	30
33. Missouri	23.2	32. Alaska	31
34. Nebraska	23. 2	32. Illinois	31
35. North Dakota	23.4	32. Missouri	31
36. Georgia	23.5	36. New Jersey	32
37. North Carolina	23.5	36. Florida	32
38. Arkansas	23.7	36. Georgia	32
39. Virginia	23.8	36. Texas	32
40. Pennsylvania	23.9	40. Indiana	33
41. Indiana	24.1	40. Arkansas	33
42. Kentucky	24.5	42. North Carolina	34
43. Tennessee	24.5	43. Delaware	35
44. Michigan	25.4	43. Tennessee	35

State Rank	Percent of Obese Residents	State Rank	Percent of Overweight or Obese 10- to 17-Year-olds
45. Louisiana	25.5	43. Alabama	35
46. Texas	25.5	46. Louisiana	36
47. Alabama	25.7	46. South Carolina	36
48. South Carolina	25.8	46. West Virginia	36
49. Mississippi	26.8	49. Mississippi	37
50. West Virginia	27.6	50. Kentucky	38
* Alaska was not included	*	NR. District of Columbia	40

come as no surprise that many overweight children are negatively affected by their body image (Roumeliotis, 2005). Many of them are ridiculed, rejected, and socially discriminated and as a result experience emotional distress leading to psychosocial problems such as depression, anxiety, and a poor self-esteem.

WHY IS CHILDHOOD OBESITY ON THE RISE?

Although childhood obesity was recently spotted on the social radar screen with pressing concerns raised in the last two decades or so, there are a number of critical aspects worth mentioning. Childhood obesity is on the rise because of complex interactions between social and environmental contexts, which affect children's eating and physical habits (Institute of Medicine, 2004a). While no one factor determines whether a child will become overweight or obese, researchers have noted two main social forces that are partially to blame for children's expanding waistlines:

(a) Children are consuming more high-calorie, refined foods (Harris, 2002)
With the increase in fast foods and snacks, more children are craving palatable foods that are also high in fat and sugar.

(b) Children are less physically active and engage in activities that lend themselves to a sedentary lifestyle (American Academy of Pediatrics, 2003)
With the increase in media, computers, and video technology accessibility, children are making and finding fewer opportunities to exercise. Children are spending more time in front of the TV, computer screen, and video games and less time playing outside.

High-Calorie, Refined Foods Consumption

In the modern world calorie-rich foods are readily available, affordable, accessible, attractive, easy and convenient making it increasingly difficult for children to keep a healthy weight. Their system of weight gain is an easy one. Children pack on the pounds as a direct result from an energy imbalance of calories consumed and calories expended. When there is consistently more energy intake (i.e., calories from food) – eating too many calories—than energy output (i.e., calories expended from metabolism and physical activity) – not getting enough exercise, the weight increases over time. As little as 50 to 100 calories in excess a day can lead to a five to 10 pound gain in one year.

The eating habits of overweight and obese children are concerning. Research has shown that they have poor diets attributed to:

Poor Nutrition. According to the U.S. Department of Agriculture (USDA, 2003), only two percent of children meet the federal dietary guidelines daily serving recommendations for all five major food groups – grains, vegetables, fruits, milk, and meats and beans. Poor nutrition has been a problem for some time now because when the food pyramid suggested that youth eat three to five daily servings of fruits and vegetables, only one child in five met the guidelines (Strock, Cottrell, Abang, Buschbacher, & Hannon, 2005). Interestingly, a quarter of the vegetables consumed by youth in another study were French fries (Krebs-Smith, Cook, & Subar 1996). The USDA (cited in Vail, 2004) has found that:

- less than 15 percent of school children eat the recommended servings of fruit each day;
- less than 20 percent consume the right amount of vegetables;
- less than 25 percent eat the recommended servings of grain; and
- only 30 percent consume the recommended milk-group serving in a given day. (p. 23)

One University of California study found that 60% of low-income families lacked access to nutritious foods. Their diets were consequently less varied and nutritious and their healthy food supply (e.g., carrots, oranges, low-fat milk, yogurt) was low, while the inexpensive and less nutritious items such as Kool-Aid, hot dogs, and sweetened cereals was consistent (Kaiser et al., 2004).

Fast Food Consumption. Fast food restaurants have proliferated and they are seemingly everywhere. Clusters of McDonald's, Burger King, Taco Bell, Long John Silvers, Wendy's, Popeye's, Jack In The Box, Kentucky Fried Chicken, and so forth can be found in food courts and strip mall parking lots in cities and suburbs nationwide. It's hard to determine which came first: our demand for fast food or the fast food appeal spurring restaurant growth. Nonetheless, we have become a nation of fast food consumers simply because our lifestyles are busy and these meals are an easy alternative to cooking more nutritious ones at home. One study found that fast food meals accounted for 32% of the total calories consumed by American adults and children (Unger, Reynolds, Shakib, Spruijt-Metz, Sun, & Johnson, 2004).

These restaurants promote and offer meals that are quick, convenient, palatable, reasonably priced, and varied, which explains why the percentage of meals Americans consumed at fast food restaurants increased by 200% from 1977 to 1995 (Maddock, 2004). These meals are generally high in calories, low in nutrients, and served in large portions, otherwise known as the "super sizes." Strock et al. (2005) noted that a large fast-food meal, which encompasses the like of a double cheeseburger, French fries, soft drink and dessert can contain as many as 2200 calories, requiring a person to run a full marathon to burn these off (at the rate of 85 kilocalories expended per mile).

People generally consume more calories when they eat out than when they eat at home, which is alarming because the frequency of fast food consumption is linked to body mass (Maddock, 2004). In short, a person who eats out often is likely to gain weight. This is concern raising because about 75% of adolescents eat fast food at least once a week (Hellmich, 2004). According to the Institute of Medicine (2004a), youth between 11 and 18 years-old visit fast food outlets twice a week on average, and those who eat fast food consume more total calories and fat, and less fruits, vegetables, and milk than those who did not. The average calories consumed from fast food meals vary of course. In general, however, overweight youth eat about 2,703 calories on the days they eat fast food and 2,295 on the other days, and youth of normal weight eat 2,575 calories on fast-food days and 2,622 on the others (Hellmich).

Snacking and Soft Drink Consumption. Snacking is also a culprit of the childhood obesity crises and it has become problematic for two reasons: 1) snack items are high in calories and low in nutrients; and 2) children are snacking more frequently on items that do not meet the minimum recommended daily servings of fruits and vegetables (Institute of Medicine, 2004b). One study found that students in schools who had available snacks were half as likely to consume fruit, juice, and vegetables compared to those students who had no snacks available to them (Vail, 2004).

Snacks have become a way of life for many Americans because snack items have many attractive features, they: are conveniently pre-packaged; have a stable shelf life; require little or no preparation; and are accessible and child preferred (Thompson, Baranowski, Cullen, Rittenberry, LaTroy, Baranowski, Taylor, & Nicklas, 2003). It is no wonder that at least 30% of the calories that Americans consume each day are from snacks (Institute of Medicine, 2004b). TV shares some of the snacking blame, too. Some researchers speculate that snacking increases with TV viewing, and TV commercials promote attractive and appealing, yet poor nutrition snacks to children.

Beverages, especially non-diet soft drinks, may also contribute to childhood obesity because they are loaded with sugar. Indeed, soft drinks are the leading source of added sugars in the diet of adolescents, exceeding the USDA daily recommended sugar consumption (Human Ecology, 2003). Nearly one in four adolescents drinks more than twenty-six ounces of soda per day (Strock et al., 2005) and as many as 65% of girls and 74% of boys have a soft drink daily.

A Sedentary Lifestyle

Overweight and obese children also lack physical activity in their daily lives. Some health experts believe that children today expend less energy than children of 50 years ago (Biddle, Gorely, & Stensel, 2004). The future health and well-being of children is compromised because the popular leisure activities of today – watching TV, playing video games, and interfacing with computers – require little exercise, and opportunities for physical activities are declining. Children now live in a world where physical activity is increasingly limited because they have:

Limited Opportunities for Recess and P.E.   Recess and physical education have taken a back seat in the school curriculum resulting in children getting less exercise in school. According to the School Health Policies and Programs Study only a few states mandate or recommend that elementary schools offer regularly scheduled recess (Lynn-Garb & Hoot, 2005). Lynn-Garb and Hoot explain that "in response to pressure from No Child Left Behind legislation to boost test scores, increasing numbers of schools are cutting back on even the most minimal of recess time to devote every possible second to academic pursuits" (p.74). In their 2000 cover story, "Generation XXL," *Newsweek* reported that Virginia was that only state that required schools to provide students with daily recess, and the Atlanta school system banned recess altogether to allow for more instructional time (Cowley et al., 2000). Other school districts have followed suit with cutbacks in recess because they also believe free play is time wasted.

The opportunities for physical education (P.E.) are just as limiting. While elementary school students have more opportunities for P.E. classes, older students do not. Bergeson et al. (2003) noted that a third of kindergarten programs, a half of elementary schools (first through fifth grade), and a fourth of eighth graders required students to enroll in P.E.. But, only five percent of high school seniors were required to take P.E.. The nineties certainly witnessed a marked decline in high school students' participation in daily gym classes, and now only about half of high school students participate regularly in some type of P.E. classes (Strock et al., 2005). One federal report found that one in four high school students reported no vigorous activity at all, and of those enrolled in P.E. only 19% reported physical activity for only 20 minutes or more (Harrell, 2003). Former U.S. Surgeon General, Richard Carmona (2003), noted that one California Center for Public Health Advocacy study found that about 40% of the sample failed the basic aerobic test and the fifth grade students did better on fitness tests than freshman high school students. Carmona went on to suggest that information such as this leads some to conclude that children become less fit as they grow older.

Recess and P.E. are critical for three reasons. First, schools that offer physical activities have lower rates of student obesity. One Cornell University nutritional scientist, for instance, found that New York State schools that consistently enforced the required 120 minutes of P.E. had fewer overweight and obese students than those schools that did not (Human Ecology, 2003). Second, by providing physical activity programs schools send the powerful message that physical activity is important now and as a lifelong endeavor. Third, school-wide physical activity programs are beneficial for instruction. The Position of the American Dietetic Association, the Society for Nutrition Education, and the American School Food Service Association (2003) indicates, "Schools that offer physical activity programs that meet (the P.E. standards national health objectives) report positive effects on academic achievement, including concentration; improved mathematics, reading, writing test scores; and reduced disruptive behavior, even when time for physical education reduces the time for academics" (p.59).

Limited Opportunities for Exercise.   Simple and vigorous exercise has declined significantly in children's daily lives, including their leisure time and weekends. The world in which they live varies greatly from 45 years ago when children were getting simple exercise by walking or riding a bike to and from school. Research on transportation modes has shown that youth between five and 15 years old who walked or rode their bike to school decreased 40% between 1977 and 1995 (Strock, et al., 2005). Indeed, early 1960s reports show that about 60 percent of children walked to school (Louie, Sanchez, Faircloth, & Dietz, 2003). By 1969 the figure had dropped and 48 percent were found walking or riding their bike to and from school. The declining trend, thirty years later, found that only 19 percent of children walked to school, and only six percent rode their bicycles (Institute of Medicine, 2004c).

In terms of daily exercise, most recent figures find that less than one in four children participated in 20 minutes of vigorous activity (Coles, 2004), and that children average 13 minutes of vigorous exercise (Marr, 2004). Statistics also suggest that as children get older the amount of physical exercise they get decreases. One study cited in Strock et al. (2005) found that younger children (pre-pubertal) averaged 30 minutes a day doing aerobic activity, while older youth (post-pubertal) averaged 8-10 minutes. Another study revealed that among high school students, a third do not engage in sufficient vigorous or moderate physical activity on a weekly basis, and nearly 12 percent do not participate in any moderate or vigorous physical activity during any given week (Marr; Carmona, 2003). Other researchers have found that nearly one in four adolescents report no vigorous activity at all (Harrell, Pearce, Markland, Wilson, Bradley, & McMurray, 2003). These type of findings lead many health experts to conclude that it is not that children are eating more calories, which causes them to gain weight; it is that that they are getting insufficient exercise (Troicano & Flegal, 1998).

Ample Opportunities for TV Viewing and Media Engagement.   Sedentary activities absorb children's free time because they are more attractive than physical play or exercise, and TV viewing happens to be the most alluring of all. Watching TV is the greatest physical inactivity in many children's daily lives other than sleep, which is alarming because some research suggests that TV viewing is inversely related to measures of physical fitness, participation in physical activity, and active involvement in sports (Lowry et al., 2002). Additionally, some research has found that time spent watching television was positively correlated with overweight (Strock et al., 2005). According to one study, youth who watched more than five hours of television per day were nearly five times more likely to be obese than those who watched no TV or up to two hours daily (Institute of Medicine, 2004d). It is important to note, however, that the research on the correlation between time spent watching television and overweight has produced conflicting results. Some researchers have found strong relationships while others challenge a direct relationship (Troiano & Flegal, 1998). These mixed results is largely attributed to the designs of studies, the population sampled, and survey instruments used.

But exactly how much TV do children watch on a daily basis? Here is a spectrum of some research findings:

- One Youth Risk Behavior Study found that 70% of high school students watched at least one hour of television each school day while 35% watched three hours (Troiano & Flegal, 1998);
- Torgan (2002) mentioned that at least half of 8 to 16 year olds watch three to five hours of television each day;
- Strock et al. (2005) noted that the percentage of children who watch at least 5 hours of TV daily doubled from 15% to 30% in the last two decades;
- Ludwig and Gortmaker (2004) underscored that the typical American child watches two and half hours of television each day;
- Biddle, Gorely, and Stensel (2004) revealed that about 23% of girls and 29% of boys between 8 and 16 years old watched more than 4 hours of TV per day.
- Lowry et al. (2002) noted that over 34% of youth exceeded the recommended TV viewing with African American youth watching more television than Hispanic and white students.

Many health experts are bothered with these types of findings because they believe that TV viewing harms children's health in three ways. First, when youth watch TV they replace a more energy-expending activity with a passive one thereby reducing the amount of calories that are burned. So rather than burn off 200 to 300 calories in a one-hour modest game of basketball, a significantly less number of calories are burned while they sit watching episodes of their favorite shows. Second, snacking and watching TV go hand-in-hand for many viewers resulting in added calories. Imagine, the calories consumed and burned for a nine-year child who is at home after school one day. While watching a thirty-minute episode of cartoons the child snacks on two Little Debbie's Oatmeal Pies (340 calories, 14 grams of fat). An hour later he eats three servings of Cheetohs (480 calories, 20grams of fat) and drinks a can of Dr. Pepper (150 calories). Two hours later he sits down to have dinner with his family – pizza, cinnamon sticks, and more soda. Whether or not he snacks again while watching his primetime shows, this child would have easily exceeded his calorie limit for the day.

Lastly, TV programs often have commercials that showcase fast food, high-calorie snacks, soft drinks, and sugar-sweetened cereals. It is estimated that the average American child sees ten commercials on calorie-dense, palatable foods during one hour of viewing. This may not seem like such a big deal on the surface, but if commercials are designed to influence viewers, children may very well seek out the not-so-healthy foods they can recall from the TV. After all, put to the test, most children would be able to find the Coke, Kraft Macaroni and Cheese, and Twinkies at the grocer, but have more difficulty locating the tofu or high fiber cereal.

While technology has made our lives considerably easier, it also bears some of the responsibility for some children's sedentary lifestyles. Children today have far more access to computers, video game devices, DVD players, etc. than previous generations. The Kaiser Family Foundation (1999) alone found that about 70% of children have access to a computer at home. Undoubtedly, computers and other media are valuable instructional tools that complement school-based instruction, but they also vie for children's free time and often beat out physical activities. So if a child happens to find nothing on television worth viewing, he has varied choices for what to do with his free time. He could go outside ride his bike, but he may be more tempted (and inclined) to get online and surf for chat rooms where he could meet and talk to others who share his interests. He could also plug in his X Box and play a round of video games, or insert his favorite movie into the family DVD player. The first choice burns a lot more calories than the latter choices, but that alone might not be reason enough to pursue it given that research has shown that youth engage in about 40 hours of media use a week, which is nearly five hours a day (Biddle, Gorely, & Stensel, 2004). Biddle, Gorely, and Stensel write, "Incidence and prevalence estimates of other media use in North American youth aged 6-17 years suggests they spend approximately .91 hours per day watching videos, .84 hours per day reading books, .63 hours per day playing video games, .77 hours per day using the computer/internet, .52 hours per day talking on the telephone and .35 hours per day reading magazines and newspapers" (p. 288).

HOW IS CHILHDOOD OBESITY MEASURED?

There is no universal acceptance on how to best measure obesity in children. However, health care professionals and committees of national and international health experts recommend using the body to mass index (BMI) formula that is commonly used to assess and classify overweight and obese adults. The formula measures height relative to weight and can be calculated in pounds and inches or kilograms and meters. Here is how the calculation works when pounds and inches are used in adults:

(weight in pounds)/[(height in inches) X (height in inches)] X 703 = BMI

For example, the BMI calculation for an adult male that is 5'8" tall and weighs 164 pounds is:

(164 pounds)/[(68" X 68")] X 703 = 24.9 BMI

The BMI calculation for an adult female that is 5'1" tall and weighs 159 pounds is:

(159 pounds)/[(66"X66")] X 703 = 25.6 BMI

The adult classification chart assigns weight status accordingly:

BMI less than 18.5 is considered underweight;

BMI 18.5-24.9 is considered normal weight;
BMI 25-29 is considered overweight;
BMI over 30 is considered obese.

Consequently, the weight status of the male in this example is classified as "normal" while the female is considered "overweight."

There are some caveats associated with BMI, which leads some researchers to question it is as a valid measure of overweight and obesity (Tremblay & Willms, 2003). Although it has been found to significantly correlate with total body fat and percent of body fat, a BMI can be misleading. Montague (2003) explains, "BMI overestimates body fat in persons who are very muscular and can underestimate body fat in persons who have lost muscle mass, such as the elderly. Individuals who are very muscular may have a BMI placing them in an overweight category when they are not overly fat. Very short people (under 5 feet) may have high BMIs that may not reflect overweight or fatness" (p. 57). In short, two men can have the same height, weight, and BMI, but have very different body compositions: one could have significantly more body fat than the other. See Sidebar 1.4. Nevertheless, BMI is widely accepted as an indirect measure of body composition.

Since childhood obesity had been a rarity up until last two decades or so, many health experts had not even considered a BMI for children. In 1998, however, a National Institute of Health panel recommended that BMI be used to classify overweight in children (U.S. Department of Health & Human Services, 2005c). Now the World Health Organization Expert Committee (Chen et al., 2002), the International Task Force on Obesity (Barlow & Dietz, 1998) and others support the use of BMI (sometimes referred to BMI-for-age) to define childhood obesity, even though some health experts remain unsettled with the fact that it can misclassify children who are particularly short or tall (Willms, 2004). Troiano and Flegal (1998) warn:

> It must be noted that BMI is not as reliable a measure of fatness of children, especially across different ages and degrees of maturity, as it is for adults, who have attained their peak height. Studies that show good correlation between BMI and adiposity in youths find that other factors such as gender, race, age, and maturational statues are important to consider in predicting adiposity. (p. 498)

Nonetheless, the Center for Disease Control and Prevention (2005) believes the BMI-for-age is a useful tool. They supportively outline:

- BMI-for-age provides a reference for adolescents that can be used beyond puberty;
- BMI-for-age in children and adolescents compares well to laboratory measures of body fat weight-for-stature measurements;
- BMI is related to health risks, such as cardiovascular disease, hyperlipidemia, elevated insulin, and increased blood pressure; and
- BMI-for-age can be used to track body size throughout life. (p.e2)

Because children's actual BMI is lower than that of adults, it cannot be accepted at face value, so the child's age and gender must be taken into account. In come CDC standard growth charts (for 2 to 20 year olds) with established curves and reference points, which reflect national representative samples, and demarcated percentiles that classify a child's weight status. Although there is general agreement that a BMI-for-age less than or equal to the 5th percentile is underweight, the classifications are not standardized in the literature (Crespo & Arbesman, 2003). As aforementioned, the CDC avoids using the word obese and instead uses "at risk for overweight" for children whose BMI-for-age is between the 85th and 95th percentile and "overweight" for children whose BMI-for-age is at or greater than the 95th percentile. But, others such as the American Obesity Association (AOA) prefer "overweight" for children who are at or exceed the 85th percentile and "obese" for children who exceed the 95th percentile. The AOA (2005) explains:

> We do so, because the 95th percentile:
> - Corresponds to a BMI of 30, which is the marker for obesity in adults. The 85th percentile corresponds to the overweight reference point for adults, which is a BMI of 25;
> - Is recommended as a marker for children and adolescents to have an in-depth medical assessment;
> - Identifies children that are very likely to have obesity persist into adulthood;
> - Is associated with elevated blood pressure and lipids in older adolescents, and increases their risk of diseases;
> - Is a criteria for more aggressive treatment; and
> - Is a criteria in clinical research trials of childhood obesity treatments. (p. e1)

Whether the term overweight is used over obese or vice-versa, any child's BMI-for-age exceeding the 95th percentile is the more severe level and should alert health care professionals to conduct an in-depth medical evaluation (Barlow & Dietz, 1998).

Health professionals begin with the child's weight and stature and plot these along standard weight-for-age and stature-for-age reference growth curves to identify where these lie in the percentiles. The BMI is also calculated, plotted along BMI-for-age charts, and referenced in a percentile. (The CDC growth charts for boys and girls are shown in Figure 1 and Figure 2). For example, a 5 year-old boy who is 46" tall and weighs 51.75 pounds would have a BMI of 17.2 (51.75/(46X46) X 703). A 15 year-old boy who is 71.75" tall and weighs 173 pounds would have a BMI of 23.7. These two BMI scores alone do not mean much until they are interpreted by way of the charts and percentiles, which can be found at the CDC website, www.cdc.gov/growthcharts. When the BMI is plotted, the five-year old is at the 90th percentile, and the older boy is above the 85th percentile. Because the CDC classifies a child with a BMI greater than the 85th percentile as

Figure 1. CDC Growth Charts for boys[iv]

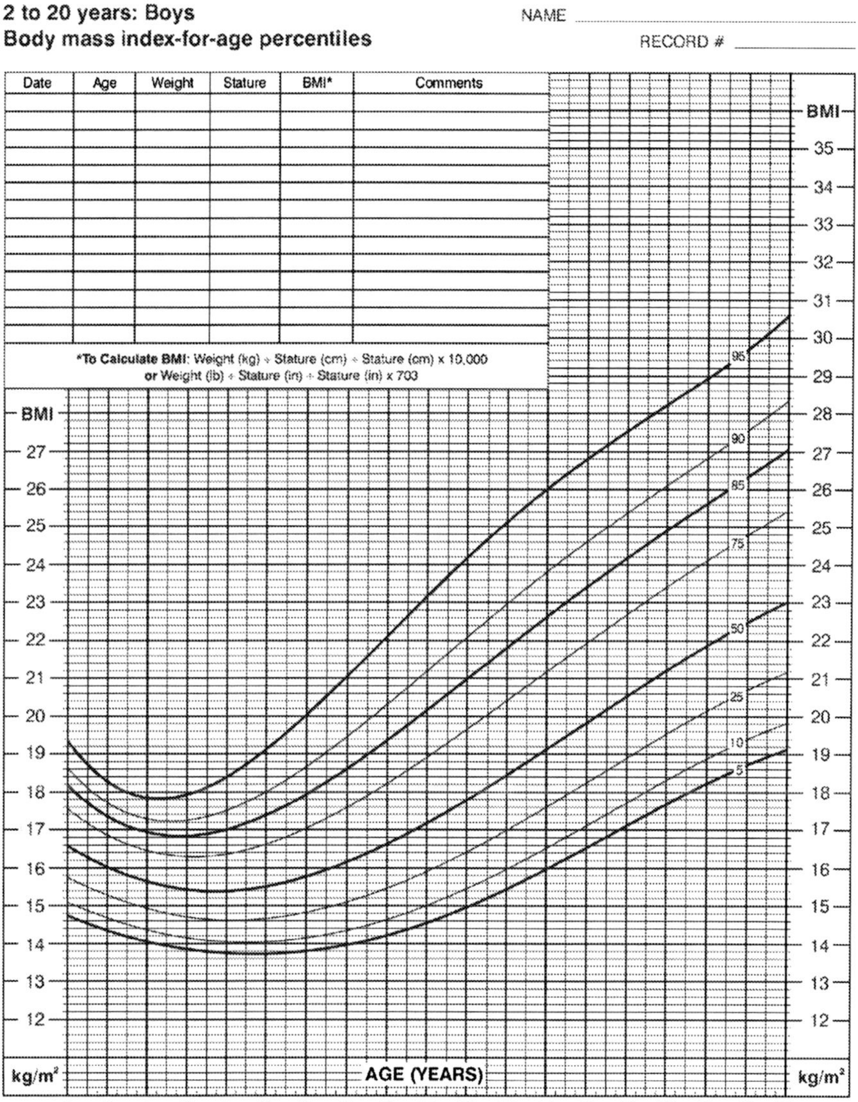

2 to 20 years: Boys
Body mass index-for-age percentiles

NAME

RECORD #

Date	Age	Weight	Stature	BMI*	Comments

*To Calculate BMI: Weight (kg) ÷ Stature (cm) ÷ Stature (cm) x 10,000
or Weight (lb) ÷ Stature (in) ÷ Stature (in) x 703

AGE (YEARS)

kg/m²

Figure 2. CDC Growth Charts for girls[v]

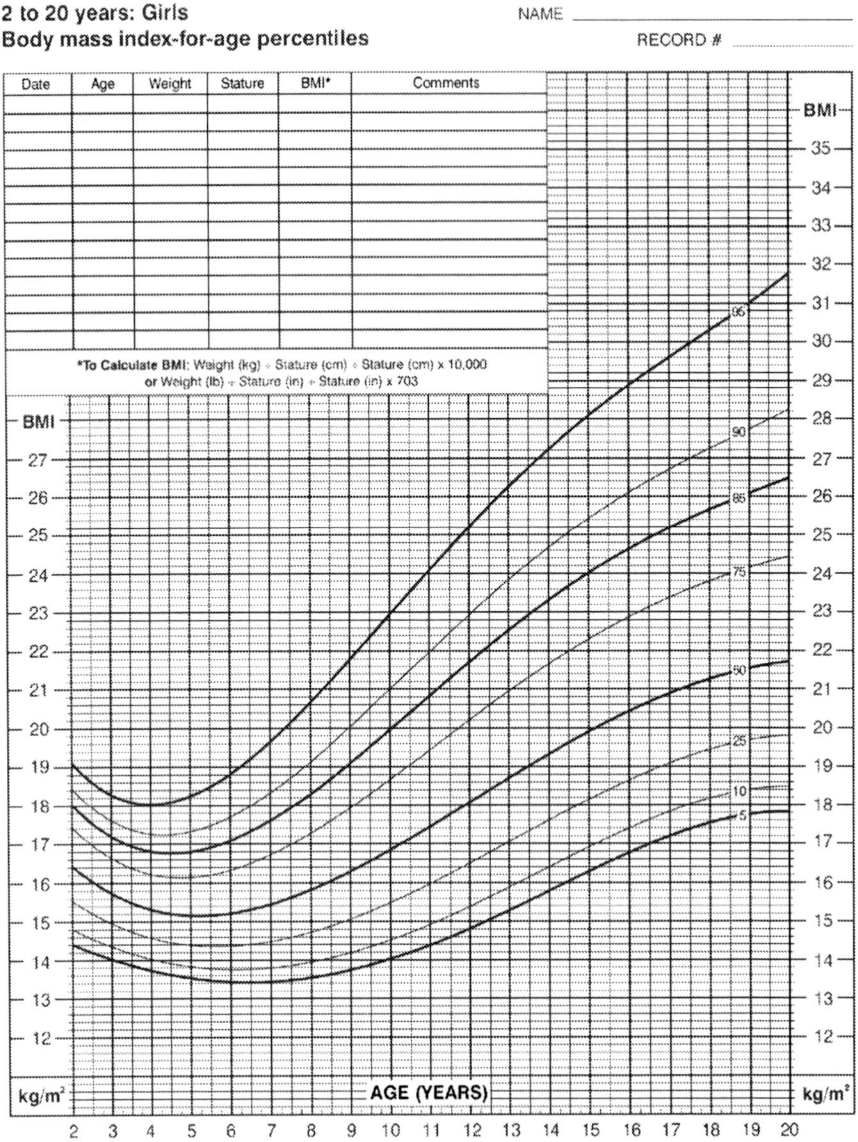

2 to 20 years: Girls
Body mass index-for-age percentiles

NAME _____

RECORD # _____

Source: Centers for Disease Control. (2007). 2 to 20 years: Girls. Body mass index-for-age percentiles. Retrieved June 25, 2007, from http://www.bluecrossma.com/common/en_US/pdfs/brochure/00-0000_BMI_for_Age_Girls_2-20.pdf. Reprinted with permission.

"at risk of overweight," and one with a BMI greater than the 95th percentile as "overweight," both boys are considered "at risk of overweight."

One other method of obesity assessment in children is the skinfold thickness and body girth measurement. It is not used as often as a BMI and its advantages have not been fully evaluated in field studies (Mast et al., 2002). As the name implies, skinfolds in the triceps and stomach areas are measured with an instrument known as the caliper, which is comprised of two curved hinged legs. The experienced clinician takes the caliper's legs and opens them according to the thickness of the skinfolds. A thickness that is greater than the 95th percentile suggests that the individual has excess fat rather than heightened lean body mass or a large frame size and is overweight (Broadwater, 2002).

WHAT IS BEING DONE TO COMBAT CHILHDOOT OBESITY?

Because childhood obesity is a hot-button issue among many youth advocates, there is growing support from federal and state governments and health welfare organizations to tackle childhood obesity. The weapons of choice have taken varying forms, primarily through legislation and health initiatives with specific guidelines and recommendations, all of which seek to transform children's eating habits and physical activities.

Federal and State Legislation

Early attention to children's health, in terms of their eating habits, was in the shape of legislation. In 1946 the federal government signed into law the School Lunch Act (42 U.S.C. 1751) establishing the National School Lunch Program. The act authorized "to safeguard the health and well-being of the Nation's children and encourage the domestic consumption of nutritious agricultural commodities" (Taylor, 2003, p. 64). Of course, innumerable other laws were passed that addressed and impacted the nation's health and nutrition, including the applauded Nutrition Labeling and Education Act of 1990 that mandated a "nutrition facts" table on all packaged foods allowing consumers to use those facts to make informed choices (Misra, 2002). But, no known bill was written and passed that specifically addressed childhood obesity until Senators Bill Frist (R-TN) and Ron Wyden (D-OR) introduced the "Childhood Obesity Reduction Act" to the U.S. Senate, and Congresswoman Kay Granger (R-TX) and Congressman Steny Hoyer (D-MD) introduced a similar bill to the House of Representatives.

The goal of the bills is "To reduce and prevent childhood obesity by encouraging schools and school districts to develop and implement local, school-based programs designed to reduce and prevent childhood obesity, promote increased physical activity, and improve nutritional choices" (Library of Congress, 2005a, S.1324). The bills request that a Congressional Council on Childhood Obesity be established "to encourage elementary and primary schools to implement plans to reduce and prevent obesity, promote improved nutritional choices, and promote increased physical activity among students; and to provide information as necessary to secondary schools" (Library of Congress, S.1324). Moreover, the Council aspires to:

(1) Work with outside experts to develop the Congressional Challenge to reduce and prevent childhood obesity, which shall include the development of model plans to reduce and prevent childhood obesity that can be adopted or adapted by elementary schools or middle schools that participate;
(2) Develop and maintain a website that is updated not less than once a month on best practices in the United States for reducing and preventing childhood obesity;
(3) Assist in helping elementary schools and middle schools in establishing goals for the healthy reduction and prevention of childhood obesity;
(4) Consult and coordinate with the President's Council on Physical Fitness and other Federal Government initiatives conducting activities to reduce and prevent childhood obesity; and
(5) Provide information to secondary schools. (Library of Congress, 2005a)

Senator Ted Kennedy (D-MA) introduced another bill specific to childhood obesity called the Prevention of Childhood Obesity Act. The bill is similar to the Childhood Obesity Reduction Act, but seeks "To amend the Public Health Service Act to provide for the coordination of Federal Government policies and activities to prevent obesity in childhood, to provide for State childhood obesity prevention and control, and to establish grant programs to prevent childhood obesity within homes, schools, and communities" (Library of Congress, 2005b, S.799). It too motions that a federal commission of health experts, known as the Federal Leadership Commission to Prevent Childhood Obesity, be established (within the Centers for Disease Control and Prevention) to make recommendations for polices, programs, and messages that prevent childhood obesity. Specifically, the Commission would be charged to:

(1) Serve as a centralized mechanism to coordinate activities related to obesity prevention across all Federal departments and agencies;
(2) Establish specific goals for obesity prevention, and determine accountability for reaching these goals, within and across Federal departments and agencies;
(3) Review evaluation and economic data relating to the impact of Federal interventions on the prevention of childhood obesity;
(4) Provide a description of evidence-based best practices, model programs, effective guidelines, and other strategies for preventing childhood obesity;
(5) Make recommendations to improve Federal efforts relating to obesity prevention and to ensure Federal efforts are consistent with available standards and evidence; and
(6) Monitor Federal progress in meeting specific obesity prevention goals. (Library of Congress, 2005b)

While there are many other bills before Congress that contend with childhood obesity in one way or another, some are worth mentioning, including:

S. 5707 RS Child Nutrition and WIC Reauthorization Act of 2004. The Act, which is an amendment to the National School Lunch Act, invites schools "to promote exercise and healthier eating and to incorporate nutrition education into physical education classes, health classes, and after-school programs, including athletics" (Hardy, 2004, p.8).

S. 908 Commonsense Consumption Act of 2005. Senator McConnell (R-KY) introduced this bill with the goal "To allow Congress, State legislatures, and regulatory agencies to determine appropriate laws, rules, and regulations to address the problems of weight gain, obesity, and health conditions associated with weight gain or obesity (Library of Congress, 2005c, S. 908). The bill also prohibits individuals from filing suit against food and beverage makers for causing weight gain or obesity.

H.R. 161 Healthy People, Healthy Choices Act of 2005. The Act authorizes the Center for Disease Control and Prevention to engage in public outreach campaigns to inform and educate African American and other minority populations about healthy eating and exercise habits. Representative Millender-McDonald (D-CA) introduced the Act to teach populations at risk for obesity about: nutrition, fitness, healthy foods and dietary supplements, healthy meal preparation, and physical activity in daily life.

S. 1172 Improved Nutrition and Physical Activity Act (IMPACT). Senator Bill Frist (R-TN) and a host of other sponsors introduced this Act, which appropriates grant funds: to provide training for health profession students; to provide training for health professionals; grants to increase physical activity; improve nutrition; and promote healthy eating behaviors.

S. 1201 YMCA Healthy Teen Act. Introduced by Senator Graham (R-SC) and a host of others to provide funds to the YMCA to promote a healthy lifestyle among teenage youth. The funds must be used to operate physical activity and nutrition programs.

H.R. 286 Medicaid Obesity Treatment Act of 2005. This Act is an amendment to Title XIX of the Social Security Act, which requires Medicaid to cover prescription drugs medically necessary to treat obesity. One of the assumptions of the Act is that by covering the financial burden associated with the medication, persons are more likely to get treatment thereby alleviating any additional costs associated with treating obesity-related illnesses.

Other federal bills that address aspects associated with childhood obesity can be found on the Library of Congress, Thomas website located at http://thomas.loc.gov/. Key words such as obesity, nutrition, and child health typed in the search button will retrieve lists of current and past senate and house of representative bills.

States have also passed their share of policies to deal with childhood obesity. Arkansas responded to their state's childhood obesity epidemic—40% of students are overweight or at risk of becoming overweight—by mandating that all students get a health report card. Nearly all 450,000 students ranging from kindergarten through 12th grade have their BMI calculated and scored. The school districts then send the report cards to parents with resources on the health risks associated with obesity. Supporters of the measure believe that the report card will bring the matter to the attention of the parents who will do something about their child's eating habits and physical activity. Critics, however, think that report cards and scores will further damage the self-esteem of those who are overweight or obese, especially those whose parents do nothing to reduce their child's weight. While as of this writing Arkansas is the only state to mandate the health report card, some school districts have decided to take Arkansas' lead and develop their own alert system for parents. In 2002, school officials in Citrus County School District (Florida) and East Penn School District (Pennsylvania), for instance, gathered student health data and then sent some parents letters identifying their children as overweight. As expected, some parents reacted calmly, but others were outraged with the notice (Taylor, 2003).

Arkansas, California, Colorado, Louisiana, Tennessee, and Washington have passed legislation that in some way restricts vending machines sales and promotes nutritional foods choices. In 2003, California passed a law that bans the sale of soft drinks by way of vending machines to kindergarten through eighth grade students. In the sodas' stead are milk, water, and juices, which the middle and junior high school students can access for a thirty minutes before and after school (Coles, 2004). In August 2004, Texas policymakers passed an initiative that guides schools in their meal planning. Texas school cafeterias are restricted from serving large portion sizes, fried foods, and dishes that are high in fat and/or sugar. Moreover, the policy encourages schools to allow for more nutritional items in the vending machines, and penalizes schools that continue to offer food that is in direct competition with district's meal programs.

New York is trying to overcome the state's childhood obesity obstacle through several venues as well. For instance, policymakers signed the Childhood Obesity Prevention Act (A2800/S2405) into law on October 1, 2003. Through a series of health campaigns, the Act raises public awareness to increase low calorie, high nutrient food consumption and cast aside the high-calorie, low-nutrient ones. The state has also instituted the New York State Action for Healthy Kids program, which is associated with the larger national initiative, to promote healthier lives through nutritional foods and physical activity (Human Ecology, 2003). Lastly, the state requires 120 minutes of physical education per week per child in school.

Health Initiatives with Specific Guidelines and Recommendations

There are some notable nationwide initiatives that inform the public about healthier lives through better nutrition and increased physical activity. The U.S. Department of Health & Human Services developed a ten-year action plan called Healthy People 2010, which was born from a 1979 Surgeon General report that later metamorphose into the 1980 Promoting Health/Preventing Disease: Objectives for the Nation and then Healthy People 2000: National Health Promotion and Disease Prevention Objectives. The 2010 comprehensive framework has two goals: (1) to increase the people's quality and years of healthy lives; and (2) eliminate health disparities diseases through 467 science-based objectives and 10 Leading Health Indicators (Healthy People 2010, 2006). The indicators – physical activity, overweight and obesity, tobacco use, substance abuse, responsible sexual behavior, mental health, injury and violence, environmental quality, immunization, and access to health care – will be monitored closely.

In terms of childhood obesity, Healthy People 2000 sought to "increase to 75% the proportion of children and adolescents aged six through 17 who engage in vigorous physical activity three or more days per week for 20 or more minutes" (U.S. Department of Health & Human Service, 2000). However, only 65% of adolescents reached that goal, and the stakes were raised to 85% for 2010. The plan also expects to reduce the childhood obesity prevalence by almost half from 11% to 5% by 2010. Two particular indicators concern obesity and physical activity:

- Reduce the proportion of children and adolescents who are overweight or obese
- Increase the proportion of adolescents who engage in vigorous physical activity that promotes cardio respiratory fitness three or more days per week for 20 or more minutes per occasion. (Covington, et al., 2001, p. 74)

President George W. Bush launched the HealthierUS prevention initiative. The overarching goal of HealthierUS is to help Americans live longer, better, and healthier lives. The initiative seeks to improve personal health and fitness by touting: (1) be physically active every day; (2) eat a nutritious diet; (3) get preventive screenings; and (4) make healthy choices (The White House, 2006). To facilitate HealthierUS, the U.S. Department of Health & Human Services spearheads the Steps to a HealthierUS. Steps funds grants for innovative health promotion programs and community initiatives that prevent or reduce chronic illness. In his 2004 budget, President Bush requested $125 million for Steps to a HealthierUS.

President Bush also has the President's Challenge Physical Activity and Fitness Awards Program, which is a program of the President's Council on Physical Fitness and Sports (U.S. Department of Health & Human Services, 2005b). The Challenge began as a national youth fitness test, but has expanded into a motivational program for Americans of all ages to improve physical activity and fitness in daily life. The Challenge has three primary programs that a youth can

21

potentially progress through: the Active Lifestyle, the Presidential Champions, and the Advanced Performance Presidential Champions begin by choosing from nearly 100 activities that range from aerobics to yoga, and then engage in the activity for a set time. Youth following the Active Lifestyle program, for instance, have to engage in an activity for 60 minutes a day for at least 5 days a week for 6 full weeks. They track their activities on a log form and after the six weeks can apply for an award for successfully completing the program. At this point, they can continue with the program and receive additional awards, or progress to the Presidential Champion program. At this next stage, youth continue to choose from the same list of activities, but this time they earn points for the activities, which are based on the amount of energy the activity burns. The youth tracks the activities, earns additional awards (bronze, silver and the gold) and can progress to the third, more challenging program.

The Center for Disease Control has also issued the Guidelines for School and Community Programs to Promote Lifelong Physical Activity among Young People. Physical education, exercise science, health education, and public health experts used scientific research and the opinions of national and federal organizations to write the guidelines for school personnel, policymakers, and postsecondary educators whose goal is to deliver sound and attractive physical activity programs for young people. The guidelines seek to transform young people's exercise and eating behavior into healthy ones by offering recommendations on policies, environment, physical and health education, extracurricular activities, family and community involvement, personnel training, health services, and evaluation. The recommendations, which can be found in Table 4, develop in youth "the knowledge, attitudes, behavioral skills, and confidence needed to adopt and maintain a physically active lifestyle" (Levin, Martin, McKenzie, & De Louise, 2002). The guidelines ultimately aim for developmentally appropriate health, sports and recreation practices so that youth find an active lifestyle more attractive than a sedentary one.

Action for Healthy Kids (AFHK) was born from the 2002 National Healthy Schools Summit when the former U.S. Surgeon General David Satcher called for a response to the childhood obesity epidemic. The response was a synergy of over 50 organizations collaborating to improve nutrition and increase physical fitness among youth. AFHK, now a nonprofit organization, works on improving children's eating habits and increase their physical activity, as well as educates school personnel and parents about best practices in the delivery of health and physical activity programs. AFHK's three major thrusts are found in Table 5. AFHK is driven from their doctrine, Commitment to Change, which is an adapted version of The Surgeon General's Call to Action, and from policies, programs, and interventions that are deemed successful after a rigorous evaluation. AFHK work with 51 State Teams and disseminates what works in each state through their online database.

Additional health promotion programs can be found in Chapter 6.

*Table 4. Guidelines for School and Community Programs to
Promote Lifelong Physical Activity among Young People [vi]*

1. Establish policies that promote enjoyable, lifelong physical activity among young people.

2. Provide physical and social environments that encourage and enable safe and enjoyable physical activity.

3. Implement physical education curricula and instruction that emphasize enjoyable participation in physical activity and that help students develop the knowledge, attitudes, motor skills, behavioral skills, and confidence needed to adopt and maintain physically active lifestyles.

4. Implement health education curricula and instruction that help students develop the knowledge, attitudes, behavioral skills, and confidence needed to adopt and maintain physically active lifestyles.

5. Provide extracurricular physical activity programs that meet the needs and interests of all students.

6. Include parents and guardians in physical activity instruction and in extracurricular and community physical activity programs, and encourage them to support their children's participation in enjoyable physical activities.

7. Provide training for education, coaching, recreation, health-care, and other school and community personnel that imparts the knowledge and skills needed to effectively promote enjoyable, lifelong physical activity among young people.

8. Assess physical activity patterns among young people, counsel them about physical activity, refer them to appropriate programs, and advocate for physical activity instruction and programs for young people.

9. Provide a range of developmentally appropriate community sports and recreation programs that are attractive to all young people.

10. Regularly evaluate school and community physical activity instruction, programs, and facilities.

Table 5. Action for Healthy Kids: Vision, mission, and goals[vii]

Our Vision

All kids develop the lifelong habits necessary to promote health and learning.

Our Mission

To engage diverse organizations, leaders, and volunteers in actions that foster sound nutrition and good physical activity in children, youth, and schools.

Our Goal

1. Systematic, sustainable changes of sound nutrition and good physical activity occur in all schools (implementation of Surgeon General's Call to Action)
2. Schools, families, and communities engage to improve eating and physical activity patterns in youth
3. Action for Healthy Kids is the trusted, recognized authority and resource on creating health-promoting schools that support sound nutrition and good physical activity

---

CONCLUSION

Childhood obesity is presently a great challenge. Indeed, this current generation of youth is the heaviest and the most inactive of all time. While it may have been a rarity, childhood obesity has become a crisis in the eyes of many youth advocates. With the increasing prevalence of overweight youth in our society, many fear that this troubling trend will produce a generation that has lifelong health problems including chronic diseases and significant comorbidities that can lead to an early mortality. There are no easy answers to childhood obesity, yet a number of organizations have spearheaded campaigns to keep the trend from escalating. These intervention and prevention measures will not curb the trend easily or without complication, but will require that parents, schools, and communities work together to reach out to youth who need some direction in transforming their lives into healthy ones.

NOTES

[i] *Source:* Adapted from Drohan, S. (2002). Managing early childhood obesity in the primary care setting: A behavior modification approach. *Pediatric Nursing, 28(6),* 599-609.

[ii] *Source:* Adapted from Dianis, L. (2004, July). By the numbers on obesity: A data bank on education trends for district leaders. *District Administrator, p. 64.*

[iii] *Source:* Adapted from: Maddock, J. (2004). The relationships between obesity and the prevalence of fast food restaurants: State-level analysis. *American Journal of Health Promotion, 19(2),* 137-143. And, KIDS COUNT. (2007). *KIDS COUNT analysis of the 2003 National Survey of Children's Health: State differences in rates of overweight or obese youth.* Retrieved June 25, 2007, from http://www.aecf.org/upload/PublicationFiles/DA3622H1267.pdf

[iv] *Source*: Centers for Disease Control. (2007). 2 to 20 years: Boys. Body mass index-for-age percentiles. Retrieved June 25, 2007, from http://www.bluecrossma.com/common/en_US/pdfs/brochure/00-0000_BMI_for_Age_Girls_2-20.pdf.

[v] *Source:* Centers for Disease Control. (2007). 2 to 20 years: Girls. Body mass index-for-age percentiles. Retrieved June 25, 2007, from http://www.bluecrossma.com/common/en_US/pdfs/brochure/00-0000_BMI_for_Age_Girls_2-20.pdf.
[vi] *Source:* Centers for Disease Control. (2005). Guidelines for School and Community Programs to Promote Lifelong Physical Activity Among Young People. Retrieved September 25, 2006, from http://wonder.cdc.gov/wonder/prevguid/m0046823/m0046823.asp.
[vii] *Source:* Action for Healthy Kids. (2006). About us. Retrieved September 25, 2006, from http://www.actionforhealthykids.org/about.php. Reprinted with permission.

REFERENCES

American Academy of Pediatrics. (2003). Prevention of pediatric overweight and obesity. *Pediatrics, 112(2)*, 424-430.

American Obesity Association. (2005). *Childhood obesity: Prevalence and identification.* Retrieved March 24, 2005, from http://www.obesity.org/subs/childhood/prevalence.shtml

Barlow, S., & Dietz, W. (1998). Obesity evaluation and treatment: Expert committee recommendations. *Pediatrics, 102(3)*, 1-11.

Biddle, S., Gorely, T., & Stensel, D. (2004). Health enhancing physical activity and sedentary behaviour in children and adolescents. *Journal of Sports Sciences, 22(8)*, 679-703.

Broadwater, H. (2002). Reshaping the future for overweight kids. *RN, 65(11)*, 36-41.

Burgeson, C., Wechsler, H., Brener, N., Young, J., & Spain, C. (2003). Physical education and activity: Results from the school health policies and programs study 2000. *The Journal of Physical Education, 24(2)*, 111-118.

Centers for Disease Control and Prevention. (2005). *BMI – Body mass index: BMI for children and teens.* Retrieved March 22, 2005, from http://198.246.96.2/nccdphp/dnpa/bmi/bmi-for-age/htm.

Cafazzo, D. (2005). *Fighting childhood obesity: A long way to go.* Retrieved March 2, 2005, from http://www.thenewstribune.com/news/local/v-printer/story/4634496p-4301762c.html.

Carmona, R. (2003). *Remarks to the 2003 California Childhood Obesity Conference.* Retrieved April 12, 2005, from http://www.surgeongeneral.gov/news/speeches/califobesity.htm.

Chen, W., Lin, C., Peng, C., Li, C., Wu, H., Chiang, J., Wu, J., & Huang, P. (2002). Approaching healthy body mass index norms for children and adolescents from health-related physical fitness. *Obesity Reviews, 3(3)*, 225-232.

Coles, A. (2004, May/June). Generation XXL. Obesity among U.S. schoolchildren is on the rise, and schools can fight this battle of the bulge. *American Teacher*, pp. 6-7.

Covington, C., Cybulski, M., Davis, T., Duca, G., Farrell, E., Kasgorgis, M., Kator, C., & Sell, T. (2001). Kids on the move: Preventing obesity among urban children. *American Journal of Nursing, 101(3)*, 73-81.

Cowley, G., Pedersen, D., Wingert, P., Wiengarten, T., Cooper, A., Gesalman, A., & Gatland, L. (2000). Generation XXL. *Newsweek, 136(1)*, 40-45.

Crane, E. (2004). *No child left on their behind.* www.DistrictAdministration.com.

Crespo, C., & Arbesman, J. (2003). Obesity in the United States: A worrisome epidemic. *Physician & Sportsmedicine, 31(11)*, 23-28.

Davis, S., Davis, M., Northington, L., Moll, G., & Kolar, K. (2002). Childhood obesity reduction by school based programs. *The ABNF Journal*, 145-149.

Deckelbaum, R., & Williams, C. (2001). Childhood obesity: The health issue. *Obesity Research, 9(4)*, 239-243.

Egan, J. (2006). *Childhood obesity on the rise.* Retrieved February 11, 2007, from http://www.timeforkids.com/TFK/news/story/0,6260,1171097,00.html.

Gable, S., & Lutz, S. (2000). Household, parent, and child contributions to childhood obesity. *Family Relations, 49(3)*, 293-300.

Gillis, L., Kennedy, L., Gillis, A., & Bar-Or, O. (2002). Relationship between juvenile obesity, dietary energy and fat intake and physical activity. *International Journal of Obesity, 26(4)*, 458-463.

Goodman, E., Hinden, B., & Khandlewal, S. (2000). Accuracy of teen and parental reports of obesity and body mass index. *Pediatrics, 106 (1)*, 52-58.

Hardy, L. (2004). Congress requires school wellness plans. *American School Board Journal, 191(9)*, 8.

Hardus, P., Van Vuuren, C., Crawford, D., & Worsley, A. (2003). Public perceptions of the causes and prevention of obesity among primary school children. *International Journal of Obesity, 27(12)*, 1465-1471.

Harrell, J., Pearce, P., Markland, E., Wilson, K., Bradley, C., & McMurray, R. (2003). Assessing physical activity in adolescents: Common activities of children in 6th-8th grades. *Journal of the American Academy of Nurse Practitioners, 15(4)*, 170-177.

Healthy People 2010. (2006). *Healthy people 2010: What are its goals?* Retrieved June 12, 2006, from http://www.healthypeople.gov/About/goals.htm.

Hellmich, N. (2004). *When faced with fast food, heavy kids 'overconsume': They eat less otherwise, study shows.* Retrieved March 24, 2005, from
http://web24.epnet.com/DeliveryPrintSave.asp?tb=1&_ua=bo+S_DE+1st+OBJECT++tech.

Human Ecology. (2003, December). Preventing childhood obesity at school, home, and in the community. *Human Ecology*, pp. 23.

Institute of Medicine. (2004a). *Childhood obesity in the United State: Facts and figures.* Retrieved March 1, 2006, from http://www.iom.edu/Object.File/Master/22/606/FINALfactsandfigures2.pdf.

Institute of Medicine. (2004b). *Industry can play a role in preventing childhood obesity.* Retrieved April 7, 2006, from
http://www.iom.edu/Object.File/Master/22/613/fact%20sheet%20-%20industry%20finalBitticks.pdf.

Institute of Medicine. (2004c). *Communities can play a role in preventing childhood obesity.* Retrieved May 22, 2007, from
http://www.iom.edu/Object.File/Master/23/369/Fact%20Sheet%20Communities-Final%20Bitticks.pdf.

Institute of Medicine. (2004d). *Parents can play a role in preventing childhood obesity.* Retrieved May 22, 2006, from
http://www.iom.edu/Object.File/Master/22/617/Fact%20Sheet%20-%20Home%20FINALBitticks.pdf.

Institute of Medicine. (2005). *Focus on childhood obesity: Public briefing.* Retrieved March 3, 2005, from http://www.iom.edu/focuson.asp?id=22593.

Jalongo, M. (1999). Matters of size: Obesity as a diversity issue in the field of early childhood. *Early Childhood Education Journal, 27(2)*, 95-103.

Kaiser Family Foundation. (1999, November). *Kids and media at the new millennium.* Menlo Park, CA: Henry J. Kaiser Family Foundation.

Kaiser Family Foundation. (2004, February). *The role of media in childhood obesity.* Menlo Park, CA: Kaiser Family Foundation Issue Brief.

Kaiser, L., Martin, A., Metz, D., Nicholson, Y., Fujii, M., Lamp, C., Townsend, M., Crawford, P., & Melgar-Quinonez, H. (2004). Food insecurity prominent among low-income California Latinos. *California Agriculture, 58(1)*, 18-23.

Krebs-Smith, S., Cook, A., & Subar, A. (1996). Fruit and vegetable intakes of children and adolescents in the United States. *Archives of pediatric and adolescent medicine, 50 (199)*, 81-86.

Lederman, S., Akabas, S., & Moore, B. (2004). Editor's overview of the conference on preventing childhood obesity. *Pediatrics, 114(4)*, 1139-1145.

Levin, S., Martin, M., McKenzie, T., & DeLoise, A. (2002). Assessment of a pilot video's effect on physical activity and heart health for young children. *Family & Community Health, 25(3)*, 10-17.

Library of Congress. (2005a). *Childhood obesity reduction act: 109th Congress, 1st Session, S. 1324.* Retrieved June 12, 2006, from
http://thomas.loc.gov/cgi-bin/query/D?c109:2:./temp/~c109NVeKvm::.

Library of Congress. (2005b) *Prevention of childhood obesity act: 109th Congress, 1st Session, S. 799.* Retrieved June 12, 2006, from
http://thomas.loc.gov/cgi-bin/query/F?c109:1:./temp/~c109AViyNV:e0:.

Library of Congress. (2005c). *Commonsense consumption act of 2005: 109th Congress, 1st Session, S. 908.* Retrieved June 14, 2005, from
http://thomas.loc.gov/cgi-bin/query/D?c109:4:./temp/~c10959UfJB::.

Louie, D., Sanchez, E., Faircloth, S., & Dietz, W. (2003). School-based policies: Nutrition and physical activity. *Journal of Law, Medicine, and Ethics, 31(4) (special supplement)*, 73-75.

Lowry, R., Wechsler, H., Galuska, D., Fulton, J., & Kann, L. (2002). Television viewing and its association with overweight, sedentary lifestyle, and insufficient consumption of fruits and vegetables among US high school students: Difference by race, ethnicity, and gender. *Journal of School Health, 72(10)*, 413-421.

Ludwig, D., & Gortmaker, S. (2004). Programming obesity in childhood. *The Lancet, 364(9430)*, 226-227.

Lynn-Garbe, C., & Hoot, J. (2005). Weighing in on the issue of childhood obesity. *Childhood Education, 81(2)*, 70-76.

Maddock, J. (2004). The relationship between obesity and the prevalence of fast food restaurants: State-level analysis. *American Journal of Health Promotion, 19(2)*, 137-143.

Marr, L. (2004). Soft drinks, childhood overweight, and the role of nutrition educators: Let's base our solutions on reality and sound science. *Journal of Nutrition Education and Behavior, 36(5)*, 258-263.

Mast, M., Langnase, K., Labitzke, K., Bruse, U., Preub, U., & Muller, M. (2002). Use of BMI as a measure of overweight and obesity in a field study on 5-7 year old children. *European Journal of Nutrition, 41(2)*, 61-67.

Misra, R. (2002). Influences of food labels on adolescent diet. *Clearing House, 75(6)*, 306-310.

Montague, M. (2003). The physiology of obesity. *The ABNF Journal ,56-60.*

National Center for Health Statistics. (2004). *NCHS – 2004 fact sheet: Obesity still a major problem, new data show.* Retrieved March 22, 2005, from http://www.cdc.gov/nchs/pressroom/04facts/obestiy.htm.

Peters, J., Wyatt, H., Donahoo, W., & Hill, J. (2002). From instinct to intellect: The challenge of maintaining healthy weight in the modern world. *Obesity Review, 3(3)*, 69-74.

Position of the American Dietetic Association, Society for Nutrition Education, and American School Food Service Association. (2003). Nutrition services: An essential component of comprehensive school health. *Journal of Nutrition Education & Behavior, 35(2)*, 57-68.

Roumeliotis, P. (2005). *Overweight children and adolescents: Screening and prevention is the best approach.* Retrieved March 1, 2005, from http://www.drpaul.com/illnesses/overweight .html.

Strock, G., Cottrell, E., Abang, A., Buschbacher, R., & Hannon, T. (2005). Childhood obesity: A simple equation with complex variable. *Journal of Long-Term Effects of Medical Implants, 15(1)*, 15-32.

Taylor, K. (2003). Food fights: Schools, students, and the law. *Principal Leadership, 3(6)*, 63-66.

Thompson, V., Baranowski, T., Cullen, K., Rittenberry, L., Baranowski, J., Taylor, W., & Nicklas, T. (2003). Influences on diet and physical activity among middle-class African American 8- to 10-year-old girls at risk of becoming obese. *Journal of Nutrition Education & Behavior, 35(3)*, 115-123.

Thorpe, L., List, D., Marx, T., May, L., Helgerson, S. & Frieden, T. (2004). Trends and racial/ethnic disparities in gestational diabetes among pregnant women in New York City, 1999-2001. *American Journal of Public Health, 94(9)*, 1496-1501.

Torgan, C. (2002). *Childhood obesity on the rise.* Retrieved May 22, 2006, from http://www.nih.gov/news/WordonHealth/jun2002/childhoodobesity.htm

Tremblay, M., & Willms, J. (2003). Is the Canadian childhood obesity epidemic related to physical activity? *International Journal of Obesity, 27(9)*, 1100-1105.

Troiano, R., & Flegal, K. (1998). Overweight children and adolescents: Description, epidemiology, and demographics. *Pediatrics, 101(3)*, 497-504.

Unger, J., Reynolds, K., Shakib, S., Struijt-Metz, D., Sun, P., & Johnson, C. (2004). Acculturation, physical activity, and fast-food consumption among Asian American and Hispanic adolescents. *Journal of Community Health, 29(6)*, 467-481.

U.S. Department of Agriculture. (2003). *Team nutrition call to action: Healthy school nutrition environments.* Retrieved April 6, 2007, from http://www.fns.usda.gov/tnn

U.S. Department of Health & Human Services. (2000). *Healthy people 2010.* Washington, D.C.: Author.

U.S. Department of Health & Human Services. (2003). *The obesity crisis in America. U.S. Department of Health & Human Services.* Retrieved April 12, 2005, from http://www.surgeongeneral.gov/news/testimony/obesity07162003.htm

U.S. Department of Health & Human Services. (2005a). *Remarks to the 2003 California Childhood Obesity Conference.* Retrieved April 12, 2005, from http://www.surgeongeneral.gov/news/speeches/califobesity.htm

U.S. Department of Health & Human Services. (2005b). *Being physically active can help you attain or maintain a healthy weight.* Retrieved April 12, 2005 from http://www.surgeon general.gov/topics/obesity/calltoaction/fact_whatcanyoudo.htm

U.S. Department of Health & Human Services. (2005c). *Surgeon general's healthy weight advice for consumers.* Retrieved April 12, 2005, from http://www.surgeongeneral.gove/topics/obesity/calltoaction/fact_advice.htm.Vail

Vail, K. (2004). Obesity epidemic. *American School Board Journal, 191(1),* 22-25.

Wake, M., Hesketh, K., & Waters, E. (2003). Television, computer use and body mass index in Australian primary school children. *Journal of Pediatrics and Child Health, 39,* 130-134.

White House. (2006). *President Bush's healthier US initiative.* Retrieved June 12, 2006, from http://www.whitehouse.gov/infocus/fitness/

Willms, J. (2004). Early childhood obesity: A call for early surveillance and preventive measure. *Canadian Medical Association Journal, 170(2),* 243-244.

Wu, F., Yu, S., Wei, I, & Yin, T. (2003). Weight-control behavior among obese children: association with family-related factors. *Journal of Nursing Research, 11(1),* 19-28.

ASSOCIATED RISKS OF CHILDHOOD OBESITY

There is great news in terms of American children's health. Based on comments that former U.S. Surgeon General Richard H. Carmona (2003b) has made, there have been impressive gains in pediatric health. The U.S. Department of Health and Human Services (2003b) reports that about 82 percent of our children are in very good to excellent health, infant mortality is at an unprecedented low, and childhood immunizations are at an unprecedented high. Carmona has also added that children are less likely to smoke and less likely to give birth as teenagers. The critical health issue for youth today, however, lies in excess body weight. Obesity, in general, is a serious nationwide problem. While some persons might argue that being overweight or obese should remain unchallenged and accepted in society as a personal characteristic (such as hair or skin color, stature, etc.), excess body weight can pose of a range of lifelong physical and mental health problems.

Health experts argue that too much body fat can reduce a person's life expectancy by increasing the risk of developing serious chronic diseases, which affect cardiovascular and endocrine health, namely high blood pressure and Type 2 diabetes. As childhood obesity has increased, so have these diseases. There are undoubtedly more children with hypertension and Type 2 diabetes than ever before. In fact, Type 2 diabetes was once called adult onset diabetes, but the medical profession had to adapt the name to reflect the rapid growth. Children may not see the immediate affects their excess weight has on their physical health, but they are likely to experience a diminished quality of life through limited mobility, decreased physical endurance, and social discrimination they face at school and among their peers.

This chapter delves into the consequences associated with childhood obesity. A discussion ensues over the following questions:
- What are the medical risks associated with childhood obesity?
- What are the social/emotional consequences of childhood obesity?
- What are the costs associated with childhood obesity?

WHAT ARE THE MEDICAL RISKS ASSOCIATED WITH CHILDHOOD OBESITY?

There are many medical risk factors associated with obesity. Studies have confirmed that being overweight or obese often leads to lifelong health problems and premature death. One study, for instance, tracked a group of overweight and obese persons for 13 years and found that they were at an increased risk of mortality compared to their normal weight counterparts (Rubeiro, Guerra, Pinto, Oliveira, Duarte, & Mota, 2003). Another found that obese persons had a 50% to 100% increased risk of premature death, compared to those who had a healthy weight (U.S. Department of Health and Human Services, 2005). Obesity is the fastest growing cause of disease and death in America because it contributes to coronary heart disease, the leading cause of death in our society. In fact, of the ten leading causes of death in our nation, three – certain cancers, strokes, and type II diabetes—are diet related (Massey-Stokes, 2002). As of this writing, one of every eight deaths, or nearly 325,000 Americans die from the complications associated with obesity, which is equivalent to about 1,000 people a day and one every 90 seconds (Carmona, 2003a, b).

While it may be argued that it is adult obesity that poses a risk for significant illnesses and premature death, childhood obesity concerns many health professionals because obese children often become obese adults putting them at an early risk for much of the adult morbidity and mortality (American Academy of Pediatrics, 2003). There are medical problems common among obese children, and pediatricians are seeing more obesity-related diseases in children that were once considered adult conditions (Heart Disease Weekly, 2004). A review of the literature finds a number of ailments that have been associated with childhood obesity. These include:

Respiratory Problems
- Asthma
- Breathing problems
- Low oxygenation of blood
- Obstructive/sleep apnea
- Respiratory infections

Heart-Related Complications
- Coronary Heart Disease
- Heart Disease
- High Cholesterol: LDL and VDLD
- Hypertension
- Increased heart rate and cardiac output

Endocrine Problems
- Diabetes Mellitus Type II
- Dyslipidemia
- Glucose intolerance
- Hyperinsulinemia
- Insulin resistance

Orthopedic Complications
- Adverse affect on growth
- Increased stress on weight-bearing joints
- Osteoarthritis
- Slipped capital femoral epiphysis
- Tibial torsion

Cancer
- Colon cancer
- Endometrial cancer

Menstrual Abnormalities
- Early menstruation
- Polycystic ovary disease

Other Complications
- Early or delayed puberty
- Fatty Liver
- Gall bladder disease
- Pancreatitis
- Skin disorders
- Stroke

An obese child is certainly not bound to acquire one of these morbidities, but the likelihood is greater when he has excess body weight. And of these diseases that restrict quality of life, diabetes mellitus type 2 has doctors sounding the alarms.

Type 2 diabetes was once known as adult-onset diabetes because many health professionals believed that the disease occurred later in life, after 40 years old (Cowley, Pedersen, Wingert, Weingarten, Cooper, Gesalman, & Gatland, 2000), but medical professionals have had to adapt the name to reflect social change. While it was once considered a rarity for children to have type 2 diabetes, children are now contracting the disease in disturbing numbers. In fact, its prevalence is increasing as the prevalence of childhood obesity is increasing (Drohan, 2002). In 1996, for instance, a team of doctors reported that in 1994 four percent of new diabetes cases were classified as type 2. Two years later the number of new cases jumped four times to 16 percent (Pinhaus-Hamiel, Dolan, Daniels, Standiford, Khoury, & Zeitler, 1996). Their report also mentioned that the Cincinnati metro area had witnessed a ten-fold increase from 1982 to 1994. The Center for Disease Control's most recent figures estimate that between 8 to 45 percent of new childhood diabetes cases can be classified as Type 2 diabetes (Vail, 2004). Other researchers have found that nearly a third of diabetic children 10 yeas-old to 19 are diagnosed with type 2 (Broadwater, 2002), and the lifetime risk of developing type 2 is about 30 percent for boys and 40 percent for girls born in the United States (Institute of Medicine, 2005). Ethnic minority children, particularly African, Hispanic (especially Mexican Americans), and Native American children, are at a higher risk for developing type 2 diabetes (Institute of Medicine, 2004, American Obesity Association, 2005b). Researchers have found that type 2 diabetes is especially predominant among Hispanic youngsters, with 45.4% of boys and 52.5% of girls (born in 2000) to be at lifetime risk for developing it (Strock, Cottrell, Abang, Buschbacher, Hannon, 2005).

Accordingly, Type 1 diabetic persons are insulin-resistant/insulin-dependent and require insulin by way of injections. Type 2 diabetics, on the other hand, are not insulin dependent but may require insulin and can manage their disease through pills, and as a last resort, injections. But what exactly is the difference? Pediatric

31

endocrinologist and diabetes specialist Dr. Ravi Shankar (Perry, 2004) describes the physiology of the body and how diabetes develops:

> Carbohydrates are digested and broken into glucose that the body uses for energy. Glucose is absorbed into the blood, then proceeds to the pancreas, which secretes an appropriate amount of insulin. The cells utilize the insulin by opening cell membrane gates that allow glucose to enter. In some people, the cells of the body cannot open the membrane gates to allow the sugar to enter, so sugar guilds up in the bloodstream, causing a tendency for blood sugars to rise – a condition called insulin resistance, meaning the body is not able to utilize the insulin being secreted. An insulin-resistant person needs much more insulin than an insulin-sensitive person needs to move glucose from the blood into the cell. That is the key defect in obese patients who develop type 2 diabetes. At some point, the persistent weight gain will raise insulin resistance to such a level that even very high levels of circulating insulin will be unable to compensate for the degree of insulin resistance, and the pancreas is unable to secrete more insulin, which is when diabetes develops. (p. 66)

Excessive weight does have its physiological effect on children. One study reported that obese children are at risk for type 2 diabetes because they are 12.6 times more likely than non-obese peers to have high fasting blood insulin levels (American Obesity Association, 2005a). Moreover, another study found impaired glucose tolerance in a quarter of 55 obese children between the ages of four and ten, and nearly 20 percent in 112 obese youth between 11 and 18 years-old (Biddle, Gorely, & Stensel, 2004).

Type 2 diabetes has not only increased among children, it has spiked among adults too. In his remarks before the 2003 California Childhood Obesity Conference, the former U.S. Surgeon General revealed that type 2 diabetes increased nearly 50 percent from 1990 to 2000 (Carmona, 2003b). In all, 17 million Americans have diabetes, and another 16 million have what doctors call pre-diabetes (Carmona, 2003a). This dramatic increase is largely attributed to the fact that society is becoming heavier. In fact, persons who gain 11 to 18 pounds increase their risk of developing type 2 diabetes by two times, and over 80 percent of people with diabetes are overweight or obese (U.S. Department of Health and Human Services, 2005). Undoubtedly, Type 2 diabetes takes its toll on society's pocket book – it is estimated that diabetes costs the nation $132 billion – and it leaves persons, including children, susceptible to a range of devastating ailments such blindness, damaged blood vessels, nerve damage, kidney failure, and foot amputations.

Another health burden worth mentioning is the effect excessive weight has on heart rate, cardiac output, and blood pressure. Basically, weight-gain increases heart rate and cardiac output raising a person's blood pressure, which can ultimately lead to a heart attack, congestive heart failure, sudden cardiac death, and abnormal heart rhythm (U.S. Department of Health and Human Services, 2005).

Studies have shown that obese children have higher blood pressure than their normal weight counterparts (American Obesity Association, 2005a). High systolic or diastolic blood pressure has been found in up to a third of overweight children between the ages of five and eleven (Drohan, 2002). One study found that obese children (between five and 18 years-old) were about nine times more frequently to have high blood pressure levels than non-obese peers (American Obesity Association, 2005b). In his study of preschoolers in NYC Head Start Centers, one Columbia University doctor even found overweight children as young as three and four with elevated blood pressure and cholesterol levels, which led him to believe that there would be an increasing number of adolescents with cardiovascular disease in the near future (Cowley et al., 2000). Others, such as Dr. Howard J. Eisenson of Duke University Diet and Fitness Center, predict that overweight children today will be getting heart disease in their 20s and 30s (Hardy, 2004).

In 2004, acting chief of science at the Centers for Disease Control, Dr. Dixie Snider, testified before a Senate committee hearing on childhood obesity that 60 percent of overweight youth are at risk of developing a cardiovascular disease later in life (Hurst, 2004). Dr. Snider was likely basing this information on the Bogalusa Heart Study. Data from the study of 5 to 10 year-old overweight children (their BMI's were greater than the 85th percentile for age and gender) suggested that 61 percent had one cardiovascular disease risk factor, such as hypertension, hyperlipidemia, and hyperinsulinimea. Over a fifth of the youth had two or more adverse risk factors, which would likely contribute to early cardiovascular disease. The study also found that the moderately overweight children had increased low-density lipoprotein (LDL) cholesterol, plasma triglyceride levels, blood pressure, yet decreasing levels of high-density lipoprotein cholesterol (Freedman, Dietz, Srinivasan, & Berenson, 1999). Results such as these clearly reveal that being overweight, even in childhood, is related to cardiovascular risk factors (Drohan, 2002).

WHAT ARE THE SOCIAL/EMOTIONAL RISKS ASSOCIATED WITH CHILDHOOD OBESITY?

Excess weight and obesity pose a wide range of health problems, including psychosocial ones. Obesity not only affects a child physically, extra pounds can also have a negative impact on a child's emotional well-being. In our society, especially among children, fat is a stigma and children use fat epithets to degrade one another. In a war of words on a playground, labels like "fatty," "porker," and "pig," are the strongest ammunition against an overweight child. Unfortunately for overweight children, they are often targets of discrimination and ridicule (Lynn-Garb & Hoot, 2004/5).

Imagine how an overweight child must feel. While loved ones and other adults may trivialize or glamorize excess weight on a child, children tend to be more critical. Take the following example, which is based on a real life boy. Gary is a seven year-old second grader. His physique is larger than all the students in his classroom and grade level. Despite his visible body fat, he is a cute little boy. His parents and grandparents dote on him and delight in his large size. His father even refers to him as his football player. Although Gary is well-liked among his classmates, he has been taunted before. In a dispute over a ball, he was called a "big hippo," and in two separate instances he was referred to as "Shamu" and "a fat cow." Even though his teacher intervened at all three times, Gary became upset and teary-eyed.

There are two emotional burdens that Gary and children like him have to contend with. The first is that he does not fit the mold of the average student. Despite our best efforts to teach children to take pride in being unique and respect individual differences, children at Gary's age want nothing more than to appear as normal as possible and fit in. But Gary stands out because he is heavier than most, which makes him noticeably different than his classmates. So, he has to wrestle with the fact that he is not like his peers. In his eyes, because nearly all of them are thin, agile, and of comparable weight and height, they all participate easily in P.E., run and play easily during recess, and fit comfortably in their desks and chairs. He does not. His large body draws attention to him. He cannot run as fast or move as quickly, and he appears almost comical as he sits at his desk designed for the body of a second grader. He is not like the other children as they are seemingly better.

Researchers have found that early in their lives children are aware that their physical appearance is important and it matters in how their peers perceive them. In fact, children who perceive themselves notably different from their counterparts expressed some dissatisfaction with themselves (Jonides, Buschbacher, & Barlow, 2002). Indeed, excess weight can certainly contribute to feeling different from others. The American Obesity Association (2005b) points out that many overweight youngsters know that their peers have negative assumptions about them, sometimes believing that they are unclean, lazy, and incapable of emotional feelings. While the basis for having these assumptions remains unclear, the articulated ones in earshot of an overweight youngster are sure to leave an indelible impact on his or her emotions. To further add to their burden, the overweight youngster can feel more devalued, or at least affected, when there is admiration for popular body-image-conscience celebrities. After all, movie and cartoon heroes tend to be thin and muscular, and the leading heroines in fairy tale stories (e.g. Cinderella, Snow White, Sleeping Beauty) are often svelte and lean.

Unsurprisingly, research has found that overweight and obese youngsters report having negative body image feelings and a lack of confidence (Abel-Cooper, 1997). Others have noted that excess weight can lead to emotions of insecurity (Mandel, 2005), low self-esteem (Goodman, Hinden, & Khandelwal, 2000), shame and self-blame (Institute of Medicine, 2004), and anxiety (Broadwater, 2002). All of these mental states must play a significant role in the youngster's social functioning because it has been reported that they often become reluctant to interact with their peers or they withdraw from interacting with them altogether (Deckelbaum & Williams, 2001). It is no wonder, as Mills and Adrianopoulos (1993, cited in Jonides, Buschbacher, & Barlow, 2002) discovered, that this population of youth report greater frequency and higher levels of emotional distress than their normal weight peers.

The second burden Gary has to deal with is the aforementioned social stigma associated with being overweight or obese. Of course some children may feel awkward about a characteristic that sets them apart from others, but not all characteristics are perceived as a stigma. Surely, some children feel self-conscious about being tall, having to wear glasses, or fumbling at sports, but these characteristics are not intense stigmas. Having excessive weight is. In children's vocabulary, words associated with "fat" are not kind, the characteristics of "fat" animals are generally negative ones, and the secondary characters in many children's storylines – the funny, clumsy sidekicks or the buffoons – are fat.

Studies have shown that overweight and obese persons are stigmatized as lazy, stupid, slow and self-indulgent (Moran, 1999). Moreover, researchers discovered that children as young as kindergarteners have negative attitudes toward their obese peers (Dietz, 1998). One study found that six year-olds believed that overweight persons were sloppy, lazy, and less likeable than their normal weight counterparts, which led some of the children to exclude overweight youth from their social interactions. What is worrisome is that research has found that excess weight is becoming increasingly unacceptable among youngsters. In 1961, Richardson, Goodman, Hastorf, and Dornbusch (1961) studied the social rankings of children. A sample group was shown illustrations of children of normal weight and ability, obese children, and those with a variety of disabilities and asked with whom they would want to be friends. The study revealed that the overweight youngsters were ranked less likeable than children with disabilities, and that children prefer a playmate that has a handicapping condition to one who is obese (Moran). When Latner and Stunkard duplicated the study in 2003, again the obese youngster was selected least often. This time, however, the number of obese children ranked the lowest had increased by 40 percent (Stein, 2004).

The stigma can continue well into adolescence. For instance, when researchers Strauss and Pollack (2003) analyzed the friendship nominations (i.e. questions like, "Who do you consider your friend?" and, "Who would you like your friend?") of thousands of high school students they found that overweight and obese adolescents were often socially isolated and in the periphery of the social network. In short, they were not very popular. The study revealed that normal weight adolescents received six or more friendship nominations, but the overweight adolescents received far fewer with three to no nominations. Often the nominations the overweight youth received were from peers who had fewer nominations themselves (i.e., less popular than overweight youth).

It is this discrimination by peers that foster feelings of rejection and alienation, which can again produce psychological stress. Research has found that overweight youngsters are often depressed or anxiety laden, which manifests in sleep problems, feelings of hopelessness, sadness, and appetite change (Barlow & Dietz, 1998). In their research of five year-old girls, Davison and Birch (2001) found that the overweight girls reported a lower self-concept and lowered perceived cognitive ability than girls who had lower weight. In another study of 1,520 Hispanic and Caucasian children, obese 9 to 10 year-old girls were found to have significantly lower self-esteem than their non-obese peers (Strauss, 2000). The obese boys of this age group, however, reported only a slightly lower self-esteem. In the 13-14 year-old age group, both obese girls and boys scored a significantly lower self-esteem than their peers of average weight.

The repercussions of having an unhealthy body image and/or lowered self-esteem is that some youth will passively respond to this type of discrimination by again withdrawing and isolating themselves further from their peers (Abel-Cooper, 1997), while others retreat to compulsive eating (Covington, Cybulski, Davis, Duca, Farrell, Kasgorgis, Kator, & Sell, 2001), which can lead to added weight. All of these taxing emotions can have lasting effects, including an increased risk of engaging in smoking and drinking alcohol. Some children develop academic and social problems that persist into adulthood thereby altering their happiness, success, and quality in life (Moran, 1999). Some data even suggests that overweight adolescents had lower rates of admission into elite universities (Strock, Cottrell, Abang, Buschbacher, & Hannon, 2005). Deckelbaum and Williams (2001) warn, "A strong body of evidence suggests that BMI in childhood is associated with various adverse biochemical, physiological, and psychological effects, many of which have the possibility of tracking into chronic disease risk factors in adulthood."

WHAT ARE THE COSTS ASSOCIATED WITH CHILDHOOD OBESITY?

On a cursory level, obesity may not seem an economic drain because, after all, it is the individual who absorbs the costs (presumably physical and psychosocial ones) associated with putting on the pounds. However, the morbidity and mortality linked with obesity burdens the healthcare system with significant costs because overweight and obese youth are more likely to become overweight and obese adults with health problems (Ribeiro, Guerra, Pinto, Oliveira, Duarte, & Mota, 2003).

Researchers have found that childhood obesity is a strong a predictor of adult obesity (Biddle, Gorely, & Stensel, 2004). Studies that have followed overweight and obese children into adulthood suggest that obesity tends to "track" or persist throughout life, which means that obesity at a young age increases the likelihood of obesity at subsequent ages (Moran, 1999; Klesges, Klesges, Eck, & Shelton, 1995 cited in Lowry, Wechsler, Galuska, Fulton, & Kann, 2002). Moreover, the probability of becoming an overweight or obese adult increases as a child becomes older. One research has found that overweight four year-olds have a 20% chance of remaining overweight or obese in adulthood, but overweight adolescents having an 80% likelihood of becoming overweight or obese in their adulthood (Dietz, 1998).

Given these statistics and the notion that this generation of children is the heaviest in our history, it stands to reason that they will mature into the most obese adult generation of our time, which suggests that the future health care system will likely see more obese adults than the current system does now. Thus, the future health care system as early as a decade or two, will unprecedentedly have to support more overweight Americans indefinitely. What worries many healthcare professionals is that it may not be able to sufficiently manage the long-term consequences associated with obesity. Some doctors believe that persons who are obese for extended periods of time may have health problems that are not reversible by weight loss or other forms of treatment (Zwiauer, 2000). This phenomenon has caused quite a stir in the medical community. The American Academy of Pediatrics has even warned that the potential long-term costs associated with childhood obesity could be "staggering" (Henry J. Kaiser Family Foundation, 2004). Healthcare spending could be astronomical for years.

The costs associated with childhood obesity have been rising dramatically. The annual hospital costs for children and youth who were treated for obesity-related illnesses was about $35 million in 1979-1981. By 1997-1999, the figured had tripled to $127 million (Institute of Medicine, 2005). Marder and Chang (2005) found that:

- Children treated for obesity are roughly three times more expensive for the health system than the average insured children.
- Annual healthcare cots are about $6,700 for children treated for obesity covered by Medicaid and about $3,700 for obese children with private insurance.
- The national cost of childhood obesity is estimated at approximately $11 billion for children with private insurance and $3 billion for those with Medicaid.
- Children diagnosed with obesity are two to three times more likely to be hospitalized. (p.1)

In terms of total obesity costs, Wolf and Colditz (1998) estimated that of the 1995 healthcare expenditures, $99.2 billion dollars was spent on medical care for diseases attributed to obesity. American economists estimated that the direct medical costs of diseases attributed to obesity (adults and youth) was about $51.6 billion, which was about 5.7 percent of the nation's medical care expenditure (Montague, 2003). The indirect costs were closer to $47.6 billion – a figure that represents personal responsibility for medical expenses, loss of income from not working, and so forth. Incidentally, Burton, Chen, Schultz, and Edington (1999) found that employees with higher BMI's took more sick days, and had higher medical claims and health care costs than employees with lower BMI's. The annual health care costs of employees who had a BMI of 27 or higher was $2,274, compared to $1,499 for those who had a lower BMI.

By 1998, the medical expenses attributed to overweight and obesity had reached 9.1 percent of the total American medical expenditures (National Center for Chronic Disease Prevention and Health Promotion, 2005). When the American Obesity Association (2006) commissioned a cost study of obesity in 1999, the economists of a consulting firm found that obesity had a direct health care cost of $102.2 billion. (Indirect costs were not examined). Table 6 shows the 1999 cost results in relation to the co-morbidities. The most recent figures (2002) reveal that obesity costs the United States economy a mammoth $117 billion, which includes medial care expenses, worker's compensation, and lost work productivity (U.S.

Department of Health & Human Services, 2003; Robbins, Andersen, & Morandi, 2004). And, taxpayers absorb about $39 billion of these costs through Medicare and Medicaid amounting to about $175 per person. In terms of state-by-state spending, Finkelstein, Feilbelkorn, and Wang (2004) found that states spend about one-twentieth of their health care for obesity related illness. Arizona spends the least at 4 percent, and Alaska spends the highest at 6.7 percent. In all, California spends the most dollars on obese persons -- $7.7 billion, while Wyoming spends the least at $87 million. Table 7 shows the 2003 individual percentages states spent on healthcare for their obese citizens. Upon learning of the results, secretary for the Department of Health and Human Services Tommy Thompson expressed, "Obesity has become a crucial health problems for our nation, and these findings show that the medical costs alone reflect the significance of the challenge" (CNN.Com, 2004).

Table 6. Obesity costs in relation to co-morbidities (1999 dollars in billions)[i]

Disease	Direct Cost of Obesity	Direct Cost of Disease	Direct Cost of Obesity as a Percentage of Total Direct Cost of Disease
Arthritis	$7.4	$23.1	32%
Breast Cancer	$2.1	$10.2	21%
Heart Disease	$30.6	$101.8	30%
Colorectal Cancer	$2.0	$10.0	20%
Diabetes (Type 2)	$20.5	$47.2	43%
Endometrial Cancer	$0.6	$2.5	24%
ESRD	$3.0	$14.9	20%
Gallstones	$3.5	$7.7	45%
Hypertension	$9.6	$24.5	39%
Liver Disease	$3.4	$9.7	35%
Low Back Pain	$3.5	$19.2	18%
Renal Cell Cancer	$0.5	$1.6	31%
Obstructive Sleep Apnea	$0.2	$0.4	50%
Stroke	$8.1	$29.5	27%
Urinary Incontinence	$7.6	$29.2	26%
Total Direct Cost	$102.2	$331.4	31%

Although it is difficult to predict the exact economic impact overweight and obesity will have over the next few years, the medical costs to treat diseases attributed to childhood obesity could be in the upper billions annually. In short, childhood obesity is destined to become a major contributor to the costs of illnesses in our society until there are successful prevention and intervention measures in place.

Table 7. Estimated adult obesity-attributable medical expenditures (2003 dollars in millions)[ii]

State Rank	Healthcare expense for obese residents	State Rank	Healthcare expense for obese residents
1. California	$7,675	27. Oklahoma	$854
2. New York	$6,080	28. Iowa	$783
3. Texas	$5,340	29. Oregon	$781
4. Pennsylvania	$4,138	30. Mississippi	$757
5. Florida	$3,987	31. Arizona	$752
6. Illinois	$3,439	32. Arkansas	$663
7.Ohio	$3,304	33. Kansas	$657
8. Michigan	$2,931	34. West Virginia	$588
9. New Jersey	$2,342	35. Nebraska	$454
10. North Carolina	$2,138	36. Utah	$393
11. Georgia	$2,133	37. DC	$372
12. Tennessee	$1,840	38. Maine	$357
13. Massachusetts	$1,822	39. Nevada	$337
14. Virginia	$1,641	40. New Mexico	$324
15. Indiana	$1,637	41. Rhode Island	$305
16. Missouri	$1,636	42. New Hampshire	$302
17. Maryland	$1,533	43. Idaho	$227
18. Wisconsin	$1,487	44. Hawaii	$209
19. Louisiana	$1,373	44. North Dakota	$209
20. Alabama	$1,320	45. Delaware	$207
21. Minnesota	$1,307	46. Alaska	$195
22. Kentucky	$1,163	46. South Dakota	$195
23. Washington	$1,130	47. Montana	$175
24. South Carolina	$1,060	48. Vermont	$141
25. Colorado	$874	49. Wyoming	$87
26. Connecticut	$856		

CONCLUSION

Make no mistake about it; excessively heavy children have a risk of developing a wide range of long-term physical health problems that could lead to premature death. Research has found that obesity is associated with cardiovascular, endocrine, and number of other diseases that diminishes quality of life. Moreover, medical studies have shown that an increasing number of overweight and obese children are developing adult-like health problems that were once considered a rarity in childhood. Childhood obesity has its psychosocial effects, too. Perhaps the most devastating is that overweight and obese children have to emotionally contend with the stigma that society and children place on fat. Children early on assign negative qualities to their overweight peers that often leads to taunting and teasing. This can affect overweight children into feeling shame, insecure, alienated, and rejected leading to depression, a low self-esteem, and a lack of confidence, which carry their own set of mental health problems. Unfortunately, many overweight and obese youngsters are emotionally vulnerable and this can hurt their academic and social functioning throughout their lifetime. What is particularly concerning for many healthcare professionals is that they are not certain that the current healthcare system is fully able to effectively support the next (considerably larger) generation of obese persons. Already, obesity costs the nation $117 billion. The growing population of obese children is sure to become a considerable burden on the healthcare infrastructure and spending.

NOTES

[i] source: American Obesity Association. (2006). *Cost of obesity.* Retrieved October 5, 2006, from http://www.obesity.org/treatment/cost.shtml.

[ii] source: Adapted from Finkelstein, E., Fiebelkorn, I., & Wang, G. (2004). State-level estimates of annual medical expenditures attributable to obesity. *Obesity Research, 12(1),* 23.

REFERENCES/BIBLIOGRAPHY

Abel-Cooper, T. (1997). Kids and obesity: Will overweight children face a life of health problems? *Vibrant Life, 13(2),* 16-19.

American Academy of Pediatrics. (2003). Policy statement: Prevention of pediatric overweight and obesity. *Pediatrics, 112(2),* 424-430.

American Obesity Association. (2005a). *Childhood obesity: Health risks, diagnosis, and treatment.* Retrieved March 1, 2005, from http://www.obesity.org/subs/childhood/healthrisks.shtml.

American Obesity Association. (2005b). *Obesity in youth.* Retrieved March 1, 2005, from http://www.obesity.org/subs/fastfacts/obesity_youth.shtml.

American Obesity Association. (2006). *Cost of obesity.* Retrieved October 5, 2006, from http://www.obesity.org/treatment/cost.shtml.

Barlow, S., & Dietz, W. (1998). Obesity evaluation and treatment: Expert committee recommendations. *Pediatrics, 102(3),* e11.

Biddle, S., Gorely, T., & Stensel, D. (2004). Health-enhancing physical activity and sedentary behaviour in children and adolescents. *Journal of Sports Sciences, 22(18),* 679(23).

Broadwater, H. (2002). Reshaping the future of overweight kids. *RN, 65(11),* 36(6).

Burton, W., Chen, C., Schultz, A., & Edington, D. (1999). The costs of body mass index levels in an employed population. *Statistical Bulletin Metropolitan Life Insurance Company, 80(3),* 8-14.

Carmona, R. (2003a). *The obesity crises in America.* Retrieved April 12, 2005, from http://www.surgeongeneral.gov/news/testimony/obesity 07162003.htm.

Carmona, R. (2003b). *Remarks to the 2003 California childhood obesity conference.* Retrieved April 12, 2005, from http://www.surgeongeneral.gov/news/speeches/califobesity.htm.

CNN.Com. (2004). *Medical cost of obesity $75 billion.* Retrieved on October 5, 2006, from http://cnn.com/2004/HEALTH/conditions/01/21/obesity/spending.ap/index.html.

Covington, C., Cybulski, M., Davis, T., Duca, G., Farrell, E., Kasgorgis, M., Kator, C., & Sell, T. (2001). Kids on the move: Preventing obesity among urban children. *American Journal of Nursing, 101(3),* 73-81.

Cowley, G., Pedersen, D., Wingert, P., Weingarten, T., Cooper, A., Gesalman, A., & Gatland, L. (2000). Generation XXL. *Newsweek, 136(1),* 40(5).

Davison, K., & Birch, L. (2001). Weight status, parent reaction, and self-concept in five-year-old girls. *Pediatrics, 107(1),* 46-53.

Deckelbaum, R., & Williams, C. (2001). Childhood obesity: The health issue. *Obesity Research, 9(4),* 239-243.

Dietz, W. (1998). Health consequences of obesity in youth: Childhood predictors of adult diseases. *Pediatrics, 75(5),* 807-812.

Drohan, S. (2002). Managing early childhood obesity in the primary care setting: A behavior modification approach. *Pediatric Nursing, 28(6),* 599-610.

Finkelstein, E., Fiebelkorn, I., & Wang, G. (2004). State-level estimates of annual medical expenditures attributable to obesity. *Obesity Research, 12(1),* 18-24.

Freedman, D., Dietz, W., Srinivasan, S., & Berenson, G. (1999). The relation of overweight to cardiovascular risk factors among children and adolescents: The Bogalusa heart study. *Pediatrics, 103(6),* 1175-1182.

Goodman, E., Hinden, B., & Khandelwal, S. (2000). Accuracy of teen and parental reports of obesity and body mass index. *Pediatrics, 10(1)6,* 52-58.

Hardy, L. (2004). Congress requires school wellness plans. *American School Board Journal, 191(9),* 8.

Heart Disease Weekly. (2004). *Study: Children of obese parents face highest risk of being overweight.* August 8, pp. 92-93.

Henry J. Kaiser Family Foundation. (2004). *Issue brief: The role of media in childhood obesity.* Author: Menlo Park, CA.

Hurst, M. (2004). Momentum builds to confront child obesity. *Education Week, 24(7),* 5.

Institute of Medicine. (2004). *Childhood obesity in the United States: Facts and figures.* Retrieved March 1, 2006, from http://www.iom.edu/Object.File/Master/22/606/FINALfactsandfigures2.pdf.

Institute of Medicine. (2005). *Focus on childhood obesity.* Retrieved March 3, 2005, from http://www.iom.edu/focuson.asp?id=22593.

Jonides, L., Buschbacher, V., & Barlow, S. (2002). Management of child and adolescent obesity: Psychological, emotional, and behavioral assessment. *Pediatrics, 110(1),* 215-221.

Klesges, R., Klesges, L., Eck, L., & Shelton, M. (1995). A longitudinal analysis of accelerated weight gain in preschool children. *Pediatrics, 95(1),* 126-132.

Lowry, R., Wechsler, H., Fulton, J., & Kann, L. (2002). Television viewing and its association with overweight, sedentary lifestyle, and insufficient consumption of fruits and vegetables among U.S. high school students: Differences by race, ethnicity, and gender. *Journal of School Health, 72(10),* e9.

Lynn-Garb, C., & Hoot, J. (2004/5). Weighing in on the issue of childhood obesity. *Childhood Education, 81(2),* 70-76.

Mandel, D. (2005). *It's not just baby fat any more.* Retrieved March 1, 2005, from http://www.keepkidshealthy.com/nutrition/not_just_baby_fat.html.

Marder, W., & Chang, S. (2005). *Childhood obesity: Costs, treatment patterns, disparities in care, and prevalent medical conditions.* Thomson Medstat: New York.

Massey-Stokes, M. (2002). Adolescent nutrition. *Clearinghouse, 75(6),* 286-292.

Mills, J., & Andrianopoulos, G. (1993). The relationship between childhood onset obesity and psychopathology in adulthood. *Journal of Psychology, 127(5),* 547-551.

Montague, M. (2003). The physiology of obesity. *The ABFN Journal,* 56-60.

Moran, R. (1999). Evaluation and treatment of childhood obesity. *American Family Physician, 59(4),* e12.

National Center for Chronic Disease Prevention and Health Promotion. (2005). *Overweight and obesity: Economic consequences.* Retrieved March 22, 2005, from http://198.246.96.2/nccdphph/dnpa/obesity/economic_consequences.htm.

Perry, P. (2004, November/December). Putting the brakes on childhood obesity. *The Saturday Evening Post,* pp.64-68.

Pinhas-Hamiel, O., Dolan, L., Daniels, S., Standiford, D., Khoury, P., & Zeitler, P. (1996). Increased incidence of non-insulin-dependent diabetes mellitus among adolescents. *Journal of Pediatrics, 128(5),* 608-615.

Richardson, S., Goodman, N., Hastorf, H., & Dornsbusch, S. (1961). Cultural uniformity in reaction to physical disabilities. *American Sociological Review, 26(2),* 241-247.

Ribeiro, J., Guerra, S., Pinto, A., Oliveira, J., Duarte, J., & Mota, J. (2003). Overweight and obesity in children and adolescents: Relationships with blood pressure, and physical activity. *Annals of Human Biology, 30(2),* 203-213.

Robbins, L., Andersen, G., & Morandi, L. (2004). What's health got to do with it? *State Legislature, 30(6),* e12.

Stein, J. (2004, November 29). The can't do it alone: Getting the whole family involved is crucial in helping obese children lose weight. *Los Angeles Times,* p. F1.

Strauss, R. (2000). Childhood obesity and self-esteem. *Pediatrics, 105(4),* e15.

Strauss, R., & Pollack, H. (2003). Social marginalization of overweight children. *Archives of Pediatrics and Adolescent Medicine, 157(8),* 746-752.

Strock, G., Cottrell, E., Abang, A., Buschbacher, R., & Hannon, T. (2005). Childhood obesity: A simple equation with complex variables. *Journal of Long-term Effects of Medical Implants, 15(1),* 15-32.

U.S. Department of Health and Human Services. (2003). *The obesity crises in America: Statement of Richard Carmona.* Retrieved April 12, 2005, from http:www.surgeongeneral.gov/news/testimony/obesity07162003.htm.

U.S. Department of Health and Human Services. (2005). *The primary concern of overweight and obesity is one of health and not appearance.* Retrieved April 12, 2005, from http://www.surgeongeneral.gov/topics/obesity/calltoaction/fact_consequence.htm.

Vail, K. (2004). Obesity epidemic. *American School Board Journal, 191(1),* 22-25.

Wolf, A., & Colditz, G. (1998). Current estimates of the economic cost of obesity in the United States. *Obesity Research, 6(2),* 97-106

Zwiauer, K. (2000). Prevention and treatment of overweight and obesity in children and adolescents. *Europe Journal of Pediatrics, 59(S1),* 56-68.

PREDICTORS OF CHILDHOOD OBESITY

Concern over childhood obesity was expressed as early as 1968. At the time, Dr. Jean Mayer, the world-renowned nutritionist and advisor to presidents Nixon, Ford and Carter, referenced data that led him to believe that American youth were becoming disturbingly overweight and sedentary. Mayer could not have made a finer prediction given that the number of overweight and obese youth was considerably smaller in comparison to today's statistics. Mayer died in 1993 and consequently did not witness how childhood obesity has become an epidemic. While Mayer and other medical pundits could have very well known the course of children's girths, many persons, especially those without medical or public health training, did not. In fact, many are still asking, "How does a child end up in the predicament of being overweight or obese?"

As aforementioned, weight gain occurs when there is an energy imbalance between energy input or intake (the calories from the food we eat) and energy output (the calories we expend from physical exercise and body metabolism). When the imbalance is such that energy input is consistently higher than energy output, the weight increases. The core of weight gain then is this imbalance, and more importantly the factors that lead to this imbalance. There are many factors that contribute to the imbalance. Some of these causative factors are behavioral, or modifiable. In other words, they can be manipulated. Other factors cannot; they are considered non-behavioral, such as genetics or medical problems. Because childhood obesity is a complex condition, it is likely that no one single factor causes a child or adolescent to become overweight or obese. In fact, health experts believe that the imbalance is attributed to the interaction of multiple factors, generally the child's genetic make-up and his environment, that results in excess weight.

This chapter explores the causative factors that play a role in children's weight gain. In particular, this chapter seeks to answer the following questions:

- What are the non-behavioral causative factors associated with childhood obesity?
- What are the behavioral causative factors associated with childhood obesity?
- Based on these causative factors how is childhood obesity treated?

WHAT ARE THE NON-BEHAVIORAL CAUSITIVE FACTORS ASSOCIATED WITH
CHILHOOD OBESITY?

Childhood obesity has no one identifiable, contributing factor as its source. Children gain weight in our society for multiple and varied genetic, environmental, and behavioral reasons, which are often referred to causative factors. The degree to which each of these factors contributes to childhood obesity remains uncertain and unclear, but apt to differ from child to child (Lynn-Garbe & Hoot, 2005). More importantly, children are likely to gain weight because of the entangled interaction of genetics and the socio-cultural environment where they live (Smith, 1999). Weight gain is certainly attributed to behavioral causative factors, or factors that can be adapted (such as children's eating and physical activity habits). But, the non-behavioral causative factors, those that cannot be changed, also play an important role in determining the source of children's weight. Some of those noteworthy non-behavioral causative factors include: genetics, conditions of the endocrine system, and race/ethnicity.

Genetics

That genetic syndromes cause obesity is a rarity. Many scientists believe that single gene defects account for a meager percentage of obesity (Strock, Cottrell, Abang, Buschbacher, & Hannon, 2005). Nonetheless, genetic disorders can directly cause obesity. A list of some of them can be found in Table 8, but the genetic conditions most closely linked with childhood obesity include Prader-Willi syndrome, Bardet-Biedl syndrome, and Cohen syndrome. (Consult the brief tutorial on chromosomes and genes in Figure 4 to better understand these syndromes).

Table 8. Genetic syndromes associated with childhood obesity[i]

Genetic syndromes	Associated characteristics
Alström	Obesity, retinitis pigmentos (a condition that can lead to blindness) deafness, diabetes mellitus
Börjeson-Forssman-Lehmann	Obesity, mental retardation, small testes, low metabolism, epilepsy
Turner's	Short stature, undifferentiated gonads, cardiac abnormalities, webbed neck, obesity
Familial lipodystrophy	Thickening of the muscles, abnormal size as a result of having abnormal pituitary secretions, liver enlargement, acanthosis nigricans (darkening of the backside of the neck), insulin resistance, high triglycerides, mental retardation
Beckwith-Wiedemann	Gigantism, protrusion the navel, enlarged tongue, visceromegaly
Sotos'	Enlarged brain, physical overgrowth, low muscle tone, delayed motor and cognitive development
Weaver	Infant overgrowth syndrome, accelerated skeletal maturation
Ruvalcaba	Mental retardation, small jaw, skeletal abnormalities, small testes, shortness of toes or fingers

Figure 3. A simple explanation on chromosomes and genes[ii]

Chromosomes are tiny structures that are present in nearly every cell of our bodies. They are the packages of genes we inherit from our parents. Genes contain all the detailed instructions our bodies need to grow, develop, and function properly—our DNA. Specific genes direct our cells to produce proteins, enzymes, and other essential substances. Each of our many genes is located on a specific chromosome. Most of our body's cells contain 46 chromosomes—23 inherited from our mother and 23 from our father. (Egg and sperm cells normally contain just 23 chromosomes, because those are the cells that join in conception and provide the baby the right number of chromosomes.) Twenty-two of the chromosome pairs are labeled with a number based on their size (chromosome 1 is the largest pair, and chromosome 22 is nearly the smallest), and the two chromosomes in each numbered pair contain the same genes (one set from mother and one from father). The changes that cause syndromes occur in various pairs.

The cause of Prader-Willi Syndrome (PWS) is found in Chromosome 15 whereby seven genes (or subsets thereof) are missing or unexpressed on the paternal chromosome. Persons with PWS have obsessive/compulsive behaviors that can manifest in intemperate collecting and hoarding, skin picking, and an unhealthy need for routine and predictability (Prader-Willi Syndrome Association, 2006). While some persons with PWS throw temper tantrums when their plans have changed unexpectedly, others become physically aggressive. The syndrome also alters their hunger and satiety. They are known to have insatiable appetites because of a flaw in their hypothalamus, which impels them to eat constantly. In fact, many persons with PWS have a difficult time controlling their eating. To complicate matters, they need far fewer calories than others to sustain them because they often have bodies with less muscle. The Prader-Willi Syndrome Association (2006) writes:

Most [persons with PWS] require an extremely low-calorie diet all their lives and must have their environment designed so that they have very limited access to food. For example, many families have to lock the kitchen or the cabinets and refrigerator. As adults, most affected individuals can control their weight best in a group home designed specifically for people with PWS, where food access can be restricted without interfering with the rights of those who don't need such restriction. (p. e1)

Unsurprisingly, many youth with PWS are overweight or obese.

Bardet-Biedl syndrome, on the other hand, is transmitted by the autosomal recessive pattern of inheritance. In other words, both parents have one gene for the syndrome paired with one normal gene (Foundation Fighting Blindness, 2006). Their children consequently have a quarter chance of inheriting the Bardet-Biedl genes, which cause the disorder. The syndrome manifests early in a child's life with infants typically having the webbing of and/or extra fingers and/or toes. As

45

the child develops, the disorder affects many parts of the body including cognition (e.g., mental retardation), vision (e.g., retinal degeneration), stature (e.g., shorter than average), kidneys (e.g., renal abnormalities) and obesity, which is centralized to the trunk of the body.

Cohen syndrome is also an autosomal recessive genetic disease. The syndrome is rare with approximately 135 known cases worldwide (DDC Clinic for Special Needs Children, 2006). The abnormal gene is found on chromosome 8. Children with this disorder have mental retardation as well as abnormalities of the head, face, hands, and feet (National Organization for Rare Disorders, 2006). They are often characterized as having inferior muscle tone or hypotonia, small heads, short upper lips with exposed incisors, and slender arms and legs. They are usually myopic and experience retinal degeneration. The syndrome is characterized with obesity because children often have an obese torso.

Discussions about the inherited predisposition persons have to weight gain have also surfaced in the literature. Unlike the disorders caused by gene defects, weight gain can sometimes be attributed to a person's genetic makeup, otherwise known by laypersons as "running in the family." Studies have found that some persons are more inclined than others to either weight gain or weight loss because of the genes transmitted from parents to children (Montigue, 2003). Research on the weight status of adopted children and twins, for instance, has found that there may be a genetic component to obesity (Covington, et al. 2001). Not only have studies found that twins have similar body mass indexes (BMI) regardless if they were raised in the same household or not, they also demonstrate similar eating and weight gain patterns (Strock et. al., 2005). A study of adopted children revealed that their BMI correlated with their biological parent, especially the mother, yet there was little or no correlations with their adoptive parents.

Some studies estimate that genetics contribute between 5% to 25% toward obesity, which suggests that weight problems can run in families (Kimm, 2003). Dietz (1983) and others have indicated that children have a greater risk of becoming obese when both parents are obese. However, it is plausible that parents could be modeling poor eating and exercise behaviors. Nonetheless, some researchers have reported that children's predisposition to obesity is influenced by the intricate interaction of obesity-associated genes. Strock et. al. (2004) write, "The most recent published update of the human obesity gene map reports more than 430 genes, markers, and chromosomal regions that have been associated with human obesity phenotypes" (17). Despite these findings, a number of researchers emphatically maintain that the obesity epidemic cannot be explained by way of inherited genes. Some experts, for instance, underscore:

- Genetic factors predispose individuals to obesity; however, prevalence rates among genetically stable populations indicate that environment must underlie the childhood obesity epidemic (Strock et al., 2004, p.17).
- Genetic factors play a role increasing the likelihood that a child will be overweight, but shared family behaviors such as eating and activity habits

also influence body weight (National Institute of Diabetes and Digestive and Kidney Diseases, 1997, p. 4).

- The genes related to obesity are not responsible for the epidemic of obesity because the US gene pool did not change significantly between 1991 and 1999. While genes change slowly, environment is a constant state of flux (Mokdad, Serdula, Dietz, Bowman, Marks, & Koplan, 2000, p. 1650).

- It is generally agreed that, although genetic predisposition or susceptibility may play a role in determining who becomes overweight or obese, genetic factors have not changed during the period of increasing obesity rates and these factors cannot have caused the upsurge (Lederman, Akabas, & Moore, 2004, p. 1142).

- Genes and behavior may both be needed for a person to be overweight. In some cases multiple genes may increase one's susceptibility for obesity and require outside factors; such as abundant food supply or little physical activity (National Center for Health Statistics, 2005, p.e5).

- Whatever the influence of genotype on the etiology of obesity, it is generally attenuated or exacerbated by non-genetic factors such as culturally determined attitudes about foods, physical activity, and factors that vary with income, education, occupation, body image concerns, age and gender (Montigue, 2003, p. 57).

In all, the best way to think about genetics and its role in childhood obesity is to regard it as a factor but not the explanation for the recent epidemic. While genetics can certainly contribute to excess weight, outside factors (such as those discussed in forthcoming section) heighten a person's susceptibility to obesity.

Conditions of the Endocrine System

Like genetic syndromes, certain medical conditions can cause obesity. While such circumstances are considered rare, persons who have hormonal, chemical imbalances, or metabolic problems often experience weight problems. Some of these problems stem from conditions of the endocrine system.

The endocrine system has major glands that secrete hormones into the bloodstream where they act upon cells and organs throughout the body. The hypothalamus links the endocrine system influencing: the pineal and pituitary gland, which are located in the brain; the thyroid, which is located in the lower neck just below the larynx; the thymus, located in the chest area; the adrenal gland located near the kidneys; the pancreas; and the reproductive glands (ovary for females or testes for males) (Endocrineinfo.com, 2006). The secreted steroidal and non-steroidal hormones regulate a number of body functions such as metabolism, moods, physical development, and sexual function and reproduction (Nemours, 2006). Accordingly, a defect in the system can have devastating consequences. Some disorders associated with endocrine include: hypothyroidism, Cushing's syndrome, and polycystic ovarian syndrome.

Hypothyroidism. The butterfly-like shape of the thyroid wraps around the trachea, often known as the windpipe. The thyroid gland produces and secretes the thyroid hormone that it extracts from iodine in the foods we eat. Hypo, which refers to "low," indicates that the thyroid gland is producing low levels of the thyroid hormone. The underactive thyroid causes persons to feel mentally and physically weak, fatigued, cold, and depressed. Other symptoms include weight gain, swollen face, hands, and toes, hoarseness, abnormal menstruation, and flaky skin (Medline Plus, 2006b). Hypothyroidism most often affects middle-aged and older women, but can develop in children and adolescents (Mayoclinic.com, 2006b). Youngsters may experience similar signs and symptoms as adults, but can also have poor growth and developmental patterns.

Cushing's Syndrome. Cushing's syndrome is rare, affecting about 10 to 15 million people, mainly adults (Cushings-help, 2006). Sometimes known as hypercortisolism, it develops when there are increased levels of cortisol in the body for long periods of time. Cushing's syndrome generally occurs when the adrenal glands (located above the kidneys) produce excessive amounts of ACTH (adrenocorticotropic hormone), which stimulates the glands to produce increasing amounts of cortisol. The syndrome can also develop by way of a tumor of the putuitary or adrenal gland, or when persons take high doses of corticosteroids to treat rheumatoid arthritis, ashthma, lupus, and other inflammatory diseases (Medline Plus, 2006a). While the symptoms vary, persons with Cushing's syndrome generally experience fatigue, depression, high blood pressure, bone loss, diabetes, fragile skin (e.g., easily bruised), and weight gain. They often have a rounded face, an obese trunk, pink or purple stretch marks on the skin, and a fatty pad between the shoulders (like a buffalo hump) (Mayoclinic.com, 2006a). Children with the syndrome tend to be obese and have slowed growth rates. If left untreated, Cushing's syndrome can lead to death.

Polycystic Ovarian Syndrome. Polycystic ovarian syndrome, sometimes referred to as PCO, is best associated with infertility problems in women. PCO develops in women who have irregular ovulation and greater-than-normal amounts of androgenic hormones (male hormones) (Rosenthal, 1998). About 4% of women suffer from PCO, but 5% to 10% of women of childbearing age have PCO (U.S. Department of Health and Human Services, 2006c). Some of the symptoms include obesity (with extra weight around the waist), irregular or no menstrual periods, acne, and excessive hair growth in unusual places, such as the face, chest, stomach, and back. Although women with PCO may have many small cysts (hence explains "poly" preceding the root word) in their ovaries, the cysts do not seem to be the cause of the problem (Crandall, 2002). The exact cause of PCO remains uncertain. It frequently runs in families, but there is not enough evidence to conclusively support a genetic link (U.S. Department of Health and Human Service, 2006c).

Racial/Ethnic Background

The causal factor of race/ethnic background is an interesting one because it could be recognized as a non-behavioral or behavioral factor. While it may be plausible that some races or ethnic groups could be more susceptible to weight gain than others, it also stands to reason that cultural differences and their health expectations, which can vary widely among ethnic backgrounds, contribute to excessive weight gain. Studies have consistently found that weight differences exist across certain racial and ethnic groups, particularly Hispanic Americans, Native Americans, African Americans, and White Americans, with the prevalence of being overweight and obese generally higher among the ethnic groups. In some predominantly Hispanic and African American communities, for instance, the percentage of overweight or obese children ranges from 40 to 50 percent (Louie, Sanchez, Faircloth, & Dietz, 2003).

The increasing obesity trend is a major health problem among ethnic minority adults, with significant disparities found in their weight status. African American and Mexican American adults are generally more overweight and obese than their white counterparts (Flegal, Carroll, Ogden, & Johnson, 2002). The problem is particularly concerning among African American and Mexican American women. Studies have found that these two groups lead other groups of women in terms of rate of weight gain and weight status. One study found that in comparison to white women (22%), nearly a third of African American (35%) and Mexican American women (33%) were obese (Crespo & Arbesman, 2003).

The 1988-1994 National Health and Nutrition Examination Survey (NHANES III) found that the percentage of African American women who were overweight or obese (69%) was higher than African American men (58%) (Montague, 2003). In terms of white adults, the proportion of overweight and obese men (65%) exceeded the proportion of women (47%). However, in terms of obesity alone, there were more obese white women (23%) than there were obese white men (21%). The overweight and obesity prevalence rate for Mexican American adults was nearly the same for men and women, about 70% (Montague). More recent NHANES (1999-2002) data also revealed high obesity prevalence among ethnic minority women. Nearly half of African American women (49%) and 38% of Mexican American women were obese compared with white women at 31% (National Center for Health Statistics, 2004). Among the men, Mexican Americans had the greatest prevalence of overweight (74.4%) and obesity (29.4%), as compared to African American men (60.1% and 28.8%) and white men (67.5% and 27.7%) (National Center for Health Statistics, 2002). The NHANES data also indicated that overweight and obesity prevalence increased for all the samples. Other data revealed that excess weight is a problem for Native Americans as well. The 1995 Strong Heart Study found that 80% of the Native American women and 67% of the men Native Americans living in Arizona were overweight (American Obesity Association, 2005).

Notable differences are also apparent among youth with overweight and obesity prevalence higher among ethnic minorities. African American, Hispanic

American (particularly Mexican American), and Native American youth have higher rates of obesity than others. The 1999-2002 NHANES data reveal that nearly one in five 12 to 19 year-old African Americans (21%) and Mexican Americans (23%) were more likely to be overweight than their white counterparts (14%) (National Center for Health Statistics, 2006). Moreover, the data indicate that among the 12-19 year-olds, there was significant increase in obesity among the African American and Mexican American groups compared to the white youth (Strock et.a., 2005).

The 2002 NHANES data finds that among female children (6 to 11 year-olds) and adolescents (12 to 19 year-olds) the overweight and obesity prevalence is highest among African Americans. Nearly 37% of the girls are overweight and 22.2% are obese, and 45.5% of the adolescents are overweight and 26.6% are obese (Ogden, Flegal, Carroll, & Johnson, 2002). Among the males, the Mexican American boys had the highest prevalence of being overweight and obese: 43% of the 6 to 11 year-olds were overweight, while 27.3% were obese. The rates were nearly the same for the adolescents (44% were overweight and 27.5% were obese). The 2005 Youth Risk Behavioral Surveillance System (U.S. Department of Health and Human Services, 2006c) (on a national sample of 13,953), on the other hand, found that the prevalence of being overweight was:

- higher among African American (16%) and Hispanic (16.8%) than white (11.8%) students;
- higher among African American female (16.1%) than white female (8.2%) and Hispanic female (12.1%) students; and
- higher among Hispanic male (21.3%) than white male (15.2%) and black male (15.9%) students. (p. 26)

The upward trend of childhood obesity is most apparent among Native American youth. Some studies have found that from 30% to 40% of the youth are overweight. One 1999 study of 5 to 17 year-old Native American youth found that the overweight prevalence was 39% percent for males and 38% for females (American Obesity Association, 2005). Another research project on Native American youth (the Pathways study with a sample size of 1,704) found that 30.5% of girls and 26.8% of the boys were considered obese, while 21% of girls and 19.6% of boys were regarded overweight (Wharton & Hampl, 2004). Many researchers have taken serious note of the fact that in varying national studies the proportion of Native American children who are overweight or obese is consistently higher than other groups of youth.

These kinds of statistics could support the argument that race/ethnic background is a non-behavioral causative factor. However, there does not exist enough scientific data to arrive at the absolute conclusion that certain races or ethnic persons are authentically prone to overweight and obesity as a result of their ancestry. Research, on the other hand, continues to underpin that it is largely our lifestyle that is contributing to the childhood obesity epidemic. If race/ethnic background were indeed an agent responsible for overweight or obesity among

Hispanic youth, for instance, then it stands to reason that they would be susceptible to weight gain regardless of where they lived. However, research has shown that Hispanic American (and Asian American) youth born in the United States to immigrant parents are more than twice as likely to be overweight than their foreign-born youth counterparts who move here (American Obesity Association, 2006). This suggests that there is something about the American way-of-life that is causing these youngsters to become overweight or obese. Unger et.al. (2004) posit, "Is it possible that acculturation to the US among Hispanic and Asian-American adolescents manifests as a preference for activities and foods classified as 'American,' including sedentary activities such as watching TV and playing video games, and eating fast foods. In an attempt to become American and fit in with their peers, ethnic minority adolescents might increase their involvement in these activities" (e5).

Indeed, research has found that some ethnic minority populations:

- *Watch more TV:* More Hispanic (52.5%) and African American (73.7%) students exceed the recommended TV viewing levels than their white counterparts (34.2%). (Myers & Vargas, 2000)
- *Insufficiently participate in moderate or vigorous physical activity:* While 26.9% of white students do participate in this type of physical activity, the percentages are much larger among the Hispanic (35.2%) and African American (40%) youth. (Myers & Vargas)
- *Have an inadequate nutritious diet:* African American youth drink fewer glasses of milk than Hispanic American or white youth (Bauer, 2004); another study found that in one African American sample, obese mothers paid little attention to the quality of their children's diet (Lederman, Akabas, & Moore, 2004).

This strongly suggest that the high prevalence of overweight or obesity among certain ethnicities may be related far more directly to their socio-cultural (e.g., lifestyle, acculturation, cultural beliefs, and practices) and economic conditions than to their lineage. Again this reaffirms the notion that the etiology of obesity is multi-factorial.

WHAT ARE THE BEHAVIORAL CAUSATIVE FACTORS ASSOCIATED WITH CHILDHOOD OBESITY?

Behavioral causative factors are the socio-cultural factors embedded in our lifestyle that can be modified. These include factors such as diet, degree of physical exercise, and engagement in sedentary pursuits. A diet, for instance, can be modified by way of eating nutritious meals, in smaller portions, with limited soft drinks, and infrequent snacking of junk foods. Many health experts believe that the rapid increase of obesity in our society is due largely to behavioral causative factors that affect our eating and physical activity habits. Collectively, the factors have paved the way for a climate that makes it difficult to maintain a healthy weight.

Our modern surroundings share some of the blame for the hike in obesity. In the last few decades or so our environmental landscape has changed significantly indirectly affecting our physical activity. Many American neighborhoods now unintentionally discourage walking and other physical activities because they have been designed with the automobile in mind (Institute of Medicine, 2004b). While much attention has been given to accommodate increased and faster traffic flow, far less attention has been given to the development of bike and walk paths (Lavizzo-Mourey & McGinnis, 2003). One study showed how people living in counties that were more spread out did not walk as much as those living in compact communities. The comparison study of people and the counties where they lived led by Ewing, Schmid, Killingsworth, Zlot, and Raudenbush (2003) found that residents of New York County walked 79 more minutes each month than residents of Geauga County (a county considered most sprawling). The study also revealed that those living in spread out counties weighed about six pounds more and had higher blood pressure than those living in more compressed communities.

Understandably, the family car has become the premium choice for transportation because a lack of safe pedestrian paths or sheer distance of the nearest grocer or Wal-Mart makes it inconceivable for some to even consider. Moreover, many retail stores are engineered to curry favor consumers by affording them a convenient way of shopping. Nowadays, it is plausible to leave home to make a deposit at the bank, drop off clothes at the launderer, pick up a prescription at the drug store, buy dinner at the fast food chain, and get a large cup of coffee without ever leaving the car. Because of these conveniences and the great distances we have grown accustomed to traveling, our nation relies heavily on cars, which possibly explains why the average American takes 42% fewer trips by foot than just 20 years ago (Robbins, Andersen, & Morandi, 2004). In this same time period, the number of children between the ages of five and 15 that walked or biked to school dropped by 40%. Any number of reasons could justify this decline; however, it stands to reason that parents are overwhelmed with safety concerns to allow their children to do so. Strock et al. (2004) explain, "Participation in after-school unstructured activities may be limited because of absence of safe playgrounds and parks in many neighborhoods. The total number of incidents of serious crime in adolescents' neighborhoods is significantly associated with a decrease in physical activity" (19).

What does this discussion on modern surroundings mean for children? For starters, it means that children are on their way to developing a larger girth since they have fewer opportunities to play outside, ride their bikes, or walk to school. Moreover, they learn early on that it is perfectly acceptable to drive to destinations instead of walking to them, and that if it is seemingly unsafe to be outside engaged in physical activity, then it is best to remain indoors where the pastimes are inviting and gratifying, but of course, sedentary. Children also learn and develop other poor habits as a direct result of the 21st century lifestyle. There are risk factors attributable to the modern lifestyle that leads them to obesity, namely: limited physical activity; TV watching and media engagement; inadequate diet and poor eating habits; parenting behavior and family dynamics; and socioeconomic status.

Limited Physical Activity

Children today simply do not get the exercise they need. The literature consistently finds that children spend more time sitting and less time participating in physical activity than children of generations past. Even children as young as three miss out on valuable exercise when their parents push them in strollers instead of having them walk. In the *New York Times*, Crain (2003) mentioned how a survey of parents revealed that three out of four parents used strollers for their three year-olds and 39% used them for their four year-olds. Unmistakably, parents may prefer the stroller because it gives them better control of the child –they can easily navigate to their destination with little worry that the child will dart off into unsafe territory. However, stroller usage for this age group is lost opportunity for physical activity that could have burned off some calories and they lose out on a valuable lesson that walking is good exercise.

Studies conducted throughout the 1980s and 1990s on North American, European, and Australian children and adolescent's participation in physical activity found that at least 50% are not active enough for their health (Biddle, Gorely, & Stensel, 2004). Closer to home, federal data spanning 20 years indicates that physical activity among adolescent ages 12 to 17 years old decreased 13% (Marr, 2004). The 1999 Youth Risk Behavior Survey found that 45% of students nationwide were not physical active enough to make them sweat on three or more of the seven days before the survey (Harrell et al., 2003). Today, only a quarter of youngsters engage in light to moderate activity every day (American Dietetic Association, 2003), and more than a third of American adolescents (in grades nine through 12) do not engage in vigorous physical activity for 20 minutes three times a week, which the Centers for Disease Control (CDC) recommends (Unger, Reynolds, Shakib, Spruijt-Metz, Sun, & Johnson, 2004). The CDC (2005) also reports that:

- Nearly half of American youths aged 12-21 years are not vigorously active on a regular basis; and
- About 14 percent of young people report no recent physical activity. Inactivity is more common among females (14%) than males (7%) and among black females (21%) than white females (12%). (p.e1)

The Harrell et. al. study also revealed that among sixth to eighth graders, boys are more active than girls and that the girls reported a higher number of sedentary activities than boys.

Interestingly, as children get older their degree of participation in physical activity declines. And, this decrease in physical activity per maturity is not just central to their time at school; this applies to their leisure and weekend time as well

(Parizkova & Hills, 2001). Adolescents *are* less active than children. On a given week only a fifth of all high school students are physically active for 20 minutes or more, and about 11% do not participate in any moderate or vigorous physical activity during the week (Marr, 2004). One study on the aerobic activity levels of Iowa schoolchildren found that pre-pubertal youngsters spent about 30 minutes a day engaged in some sort of aerobic activity, while the post-pubertal youth averaged around 8 to ten minutes (Strock et al [look for at PCL c/17/19]. Another study found that 69% of high school freshman participate in vigorous physical activity regularly, but only 55% of high school seniors engage in the same degree of activity (Grunbaum, et. al., 2003). And, of 12 to 13 year-olds, 69% participate in some form of regular physical activity. But the figure is closer to 38% for young adults (Thompson & Shanley, 2004). The statistics are particularly chilling for girls. Reportedly, data on nine to 18 year-old girls reveal that as they age there is a 35% decline in daily physical activity for white girls and an 83% decline for African American girls (Dalton, 2004).

Conceivably, the younger children have more opportunities for physical exercise because they are more likely to have recess, physical education programs, and organized sports at hand. The older youth, however, are more limited in terms of their physical activity outlets. Recess is unheard of in high school, and there is no assurance that physical education will be required for all four years. Of course, organized sports are an option, but not all students can make the high school team cut. Thompson and Shanley (2004) underscore, "Most teens who participate in team sports get the recommended 60 minutes per day of physical activity. Unfortunately, only a select group of kids go out for and are chosen to play on their school sport teams. Once kids enter middle and high school, it is more difficult to make the teams and to participate regularly in sports" (p. 88).

Particularly worrisome is the weakening of physical education (PE) programs in our nation's schools. Although the leading objective of Healthy People 2010 is to engage all people (including children) in regular physical activity, PE is vanishing from our nation's schools and the number of students participating in school-based PE programs is declining (Yackel, 2003). Datar and Sturm (2004) write, "Although guidelines recommend that students have daily classes, receive a substantial percentage of their weekly amount of in-school physical activity in PE classes, and be physically active for at least half of the PE class time, only a small minority of children have daily classes, and active class time is far below 50%" (1501). Adolescents do not fare better. During the 1990s, the percentage of high school students participating in daily PE dropped from 42% to 28% (Centers for Disease Control and Prevention). In 2003, a little over half of high school students participated in some form of PE on a regular basis (National Association for Sport and Physical Education, 2006). Accordingly, 71% of freshman, 61% of sophomores, 46% of juniors, and 40% of seniors were enrolled in PE.

Most persons are surprised to learn that there is no federal mandate for PE. States determine the minimum PE requirements without any incentives from the federal government, and they in turn empower local school districts to decide the PE requisites. Consequently, there is almost no consistency among states and school districts in how PE is mandated, which explains why PE varies among districts, schools, and grade levels. Burgeson et. al. (2001) discovered that 8% of elementary schools, 6.4% of middle or junior high schools, and 5.8% of high schools offered a daily PE program for the entire student body, for the full school year. In terms of state mandates, in 2006:

- 36 states required PE for elementary aged students, and of these 100% was required for children in first through 5th grade and 94% was required for 6th graders;
- 33 states required PE for middle/junior high students, and of these 91% was required for adolescents in 7th grade and 85% in 8th grade;
- 42 states required PE for high school students, and of these 76% did not specify the grade PE must be taken; and
- The majority of states did not mandate a prescribed number of minutes of physical education per week. (National Association for Sport and Physical Education, 2006)

Consult Table 8 for a glimpse of the states that mandate PE for elementary, middle/junior high, and high schools.

Finding such as these has led the National Association for Sport and Physical Education (2006) to write in their comprehensive report, *Shape of the Nation*:

Twenty years after the U.S. Congress passed House Concurrent Resolution 97 encouraging state and local governments and local education agencies to provide high-quality daily physical education programs for all children in kindergarten through grade 12; 15 years after Goals 2o0 called for inclusion of physical education as an integral component of all school programs; and five years after the *Surgeon General's Call to Action to Prevent and Decrease Overweight and Obesity* put forth daily K-12 physical education for all children as a key action, inadequate progress has been made. (p. 6)

TV Watching and Media Engagement

TV is responsible for much of today's sedentary lifestyle. Watching TV is a popular pastime among youth and adults alike and has become increasingly so since the first broadcast program aired in the 1950s. In fact, one study revealed that TV watching was among the top five leisure activities most popular among third and fourth grade boys and girls (Harrell, Gansky, Bradley, & McMurray, 1997). By no surprise has research found that children and youth between two and 17 years old spend about three years of their waking lives watching TV (Robinson, 1998). Ergo, much of the literature on physical inactivity inevitably includes a discourse on TV watching as a causative factor of overweight and obesity because it displaces opportunities for youth to exercise or be active. In short, watching TV, either broadcast programs or DVD/videos, is time spent sitting and burning few calories.

There is certainly no harm when a child watches TV for an hour or two each day, but when it exceeds three to four hours, concern should set in, especially since

Table 9. State physical education practices

States that Mandate Elementary School PE

Alabama	Kansas	Nebraska	Rhode Island
Arkansas	Louisiana	New	South
California	Maine	Hampshire	Carolina
District of	Maryland	New Jersey	Tennessee
Columbia	Massachusetts	New Mexico	Utah
Delaware	Minnesota	New York	Virginia
Georgia	Mississippi	North	Vermont
Hawaii	Missouri	Carolina	Washington
Idaho	Montana	Ohio	West Virginia
Illinois		Oklahoma	Wisconsin
		Pennsylvania	

States that Mandate Middle/Junior High School PE

Alabama	Maryland	New Jersey	Utah
Arkansas	Massachusetts	New Mexico	Virginia
California	Minnesota	New York	Vermont
District of	Mississippi	North	Washington
Columbia	Missouri	Carolina	West Virginia
Delaware	Montana	Ohio	Wisconsin
Idaho	Nebraska	Pennsylvania	
Illinois	Nevada	Rhode Island	
Louisiana	New	South	
Maine	Hampshire	Carolina	
		Tennessee	

States that Mandate High School PE

Alabama	Indiana	Nevada	South
Arizona	Iowa	New	Dakota
Arkansas	Kansas	Hampshire	Tennessee
California	Kentucky	New Jersey	Texas
Connecticut	Louisiana	New Mexico	Utah
District of	Maine	New York	Virginia
Columbia	Maryland	North	Vermont
Delaware	Massachusetts	Carolina	Washington
Florida	Minnesota	Ohio	West
Georgia	Missouri	Oregon	Virginia
Hawaii	Montana	Pennsylvania	Wisconsin
Illinois		Rhode Island	
		South	
		Carolina	

research has established a link between childhood obesity and hours spent watching TV (Matheson, Killen, Wang, Varady, & Robinson, 2004). The first comprehensive study on American children, their TV consumption, and its association with body weight was published in 1985. Dietz and Gortmaker (1985) analyzed data on more than 13,000 children and found correlation between the amount of time they spent watching TV and the prevalence of obesity. In particular, the prevalence of obesity increased 2% for each additional hour of TV the sample watched even when other variables were controlled. Since then others have supported the notion that the risk of becoming overweight or obese increases as the number of hours spent watching TV increases. Alternately, research has shown that the lowest prevalence of obesity is seen in the population of children who watch less than two hours of TV (Gortmaker, Must, Sobol, Peterson, Colditz, & Dietz, 1996).

Extensive TV watching is unhealthy for children for a variety reasons. Youth who live a TV-centered life:

Expend very little energy as they gaze upon the screen. Watching TV is considered one of the slowest metabolic rates around. Some authors have found that sleeping, reading, and doing homework burns off more calories than watching TV (Klesges, Shelton, & Lesges, 1993 cited in Clocksin, Watson, & Ransdell, 2002), although others have not found notable differences in metabolic rates between TV watching and other sedentary activities (Storey, Forshee, Weaver, & Sansalone, 2003). Nonetheless, TV is a poor substitute for active play and exercise.

Are exposed to food commercials and advertisements that influence them to purchase and eat high-calorie foods that are low in nutrients. It is not coincidence that commercials of processed foods such as sweetened cereals, candies, chips, soft drinks, and other energy-dense snacks abound during popular kid shows. It is a marketing genius. The food giants target youth to promote their products by way of imaginative characters, comical scenes, catchy phrases, and powerful adjectives to depict a palatable product. Within time and overexposure of products such as Kraft Macaroni & Cheese, Oreos, or Cheetohs, children can easily identify them and begin to beg their parents for brand name foods. (After all, how many children could identify a brand of tofu or edamame?) Given that children see about ten commercials per hour that promote processed foods (including fast foods), in a year's time they are bombarded with nearly 40,000 of ads that drive them to consume products that lead to weight gain (Kaiser Family Foundation, 2004). The number of new food products advertised to children is growing. Between 1994 and 2004 the number of new foods targeted to children grew from 52 to 500 (Egan, 2005). The amount of money food giants spend on advertising is enormous. The Institute of Medicine (2004a) reports:

> Food and beverage advertisers collectively spend $10 billion to $12 billion a year to reach children and youth. Of that, more than $1 billion is spent on media advertising to children, that reaches them primarily through television; more than $4.5 billion is spent on youth-targeted promotions such as premiums, coupons, sweepstakes, and contests; $2 billion is spent on youth-targeted public relations; and $3 billion is spent on packaging designed for children. (p.1)

Additionally, some food giants intentionally employ popular cartoon and movie characters to make their products metaphorically appetizing. Because in the minds of many children who do not have the cognitive ability to distinguish when they are being informed from when they are being lured, a product must be good and good for you if the cartoon character they hold in high esteem is positioned near the label they are endorsing.

Snack on high-calorie, low nutrient foods while watching TV.   It is quite common in our society to eat as we watch TV. In fact, it has become a way of life. While snacking may seem like a harmless habit, it is the source of added calories that can lead to weight gain, especially when it is excessive. And youth who watch a lot of TV snack too often. A Stanford University study on the TV viewing and eating habits of third and fifth grade students found that children consume nearly 18% of the daily calories in front of the TV, and the figure jumps to 26% on the weekends – clearly a quarter of their diet is consumed while watching TV (Matheson, Killen, Wang, Varady, & Robinson, 2004). The researchers also noted that snacking was most frequent when they watched TV, and that children ate fewer vegetables when the TV was on. Others have also found that TV viewing increases dietary intake that is nutritionally inferior (Robinson & Killen, 1995; Robinson, 2001; Dietz & Gortmaker, 1985, Dennison, Erb, & Jenkins, 2002). In short, increased TV viewing is associated with potentially unhealthy dietary practices (Lowry, Weschler, Galuska, Fulton, & Kann, 2002).

Aside from the fact that the number of reported hours that children and adolescents watch TV varies according to research, the findings are consistent: American children and youth watch a lot of TV and have consistently for decades. Research in the 1950s (Himmelweit et al. 1958), 1960s (Schramm et al., 1961), and 1970s (Lyle & Hoffman, 1972; Greenberg, 1976) (D/B1/9) revealed that earlier generations of youth, particularly 11 to 17 year-olds watched about 3.1 hours of TV per day, which is consistent with current figures (Marr, 2004). The average young person today continues to watch more than the recommended one two hours per day (American Academy of Pediatrics, 2001). Here is a glimpse of some research results:

- The population of two to 11 year olds watch about 23 hours of TV per week (Drohan, 2002);
- Over a quarter of eight to 16 year olds watched at least 4 hours of TV per day (Anderson, Crespo, Bartlett, Cheskin, & Pratt, 1998)
- The average child watches two and a half hours of TV per day, which is 10 times more than what they devote to vigorous physical activity (Ludwig & Gortmaker, 2004);
- On average, 43% of children watch more than two hours of TV per school day; TV watching is greatest among African American (74%) youth followed by Hispanic (52%) and white (34%) youngsters (Lowry, Wechslher, Galuska, Fulton, & Kann, 2002);
- The percentage of youth who spend at least five hours per day watching TV increased from 15% to 30% in the last twenty years (C/17/19);

- Children two to five years-old watched an average of 18.2 hours of TV per week (Stanger, 1998); and
- About a quarter of one year-olds and 57% of four year-olds watch more than two hours of TV per day (Dennison, Erb, & Jenkins, 2002).

Given that TV watching is far from being an intense calorie-burning activity, it should come as very little surprise that researchers have detected a close association between watching TV and being overweight (Crespo & Arbesman, 2003). Some studies suggest that children who watch over four hours of TV per day have increased BMI's. In fact, youth who watched more than five hours of TV per day were nearly four and half times more likely to be overweight than their counterparts who watch no TV or up to two hours daily (Gortmaker, Must, Sobol, Peterson, Colditz, & Dietz, 1996). Preschool youngsters are not immune from this occurrence. One particular study found that preschoolers who had a TV in their bedroom watched more TV and were more likely to be overweight than their counterparts who did not (Dennison, Erb, & Jenkins, 2002). What is particularly striking is that the study found that 40% of preschool children had a TV in their bedroom. Other studies have produced similar findings for older youth with as many as a third who have a TV in the bedroom. One California survey, for instance, indicated that 38% of one to four year olds and 43% of third and fourth graders had a TV in their bedroom (Robinson, 1999). The figure was closer to 54% for the sixth and seventh graders in a Boston study (Weicha, Sobol, Peterson, & Gortmaker, 2001). A more recent study found that 63% of children between six and 13 had a television set in their bedroom (Jordan, Hersey, McDivitt, & Heitler, 2006). These figures concurrently suggest that having a TV in the bedroom is commonplace and a fundamental ingredient of the recipe for weight gain.

Engaging in media is also a factor that leads some children to gain weight. Playing video games, using the computer, surfing the web, or talking on the cell phone contributes to the modern sedentary lifestyle. Today's youth spend a lot of time with their eyes fixed on a screen. The average American youth spends nearly a fulltime workweek using media (Rideout, Foehr, Roberts, & Brodie, 1999). Former U.S. Surgeon General Richard Carmona (2003) has even emphasized that it looks like the latest generation of youth spend more time engaged in media than in playgrounds nationwide, and the Kaiser Family Foundation (2004) stresses that children today spend more time engaged in media than doing anything else besides sleeping. That our youth are overwhelmingly occupied with media is unsettling because the amount of exercise involved in typing on the keyboard and jerking a joystick is minimal, and a daily dose of inadequate exercise is sure to lead to weight gain (Proctor, Moore, Gao, Cupples, Bradlee, Hood, & Ellison, 2003).

The advances in media have become an attractive invitation for children and adolescents to spend increasing amounts of time using them, not to mention that DVDs, video games, computer software, and the Internet is readily accessible. One study has already found a 6% growth in children's use of media from 1999 to 2000. Late 1990s data indicated that on average 6 to 17 year-olds each day spent about .63 hours playing videos and .77 hours using the computer (D/B1/9 you need to find at UIW) (Stanger, 1997, 1998; Stanger & Gridina, 1999; Woodward & Gridina, 2000). But data from a recent study found that:

- Six to seven year olds spend about 51 minutes playing video games, and 14 minutes using the computer;
- Nine to 10 year olds spend about one hour and 34 minutes playing video games, and 51 minutes using the computer; and
- 12 to 13 year olds spend about one hour and 49 minutes playing video games, and hour and 19 minutes using the computer. (Jordan, Hersey, McDivitt, Heitzler, 2006)

The same 2006 study revealed that families on average had four working TVs in their homes. Almost all them had at least a VCR or DVD player, 88% had a video game unit, 85% had a computer, and 56% had Internet access. Contrasted with earlier data, where almost half of American families owned all four media hardware (TV, VCR, video game unit, and computer) in 2000, which was up from a third of families in 1997, it is evident that media and media use is becoming a permanent fixture in home across the nation (D/7/259 you need to find in Marr, 2004).

Inadequate Diet and Poor Eating Habits

A repeated pattern throughout this text is that diet quality affects health. In short, a consistently inadequate diet of foods that are high in fat and calorie-packed can lead to weight gain. Equally apparent is that these types of foods are readily available, appetizing, and inexpensive, which has incited an increasing number of Americans to choose these over healthier foods. This recent social phenomena has led the Center for Disease Control to publicly emphasize that unhealthy dietary behaviors are associated with the leading cause of mortality and morbidity among all age groups (Massey-Stokes, 2002). Moreover, Healthy People 2010 (U.S. Department of Health & Human Services, 2006b) promotes good nutrition as a priority to improve health and quality of life. See Table 10 for some of the nutrition objectives for children and adolescents.

Poor dietary practices is concerning because inferior nutritional intake can hinder the growth and development of youth (Neumark-Sztainer, Story, Hannan, & Croll, 2002). Just as critical is the notion that poor eating habits in youth can pave the way for poor eating habits in adulthood. Thus far, research has established that the dietary behavior of youth today is one that has veered from healthier foods to nutrient low ones, which are often fast and processed foods. Indeed, Americans spend more money on fast foods than ever before. When John F. Kennedy was president, about 20% of an American's food dollar was spent on fast food. Today, that figure is closer to 50% (Louie, Sanchez, Faircloth, & Dietz, 2003). Maddock (2004) has even noted that the percentage of meals consumed at fast food restaurants increased by 200% from 1977 to 1995, reflecting the rise in obesity. During this time the portion sizes of fast food meals have also gotten bigger. Maddock indicated that in a ten-year period (1988-1998) the portion sizes of

Table 10. Some Healthy 2010 nutrition objectives for children and adolescents[iii]

- Increase the proportion of persons aged 2 years and older who consume at least two daily servings of fruit.
- Increase the proportion of persons aged 2 years and older who consume at least three daily servings of vegetables, with at least one-third being dark green or orange vegetable.
- Increase the proportion of persons aged 2 years and older who consume at least six daily servings of grain products, with at least three being whole grains.
- Increase the proportion of persons aged 2 years and older who consume no more than 30 percent of calories from total fat
- Increase the proportion of persons aged 2 years and older who consume 2,400 mg or less of sodium daily.
- Increase the proportion of persons aged 2 years and older who meet dietary recommendations for calcium.
- Increase the proportion of children and adolescents aged 6 to 19 years whose intake of meals and snacks at school contributes to good overall dietary quality.

hamburgers increased by 97 kcal, French fries by 68 kcal, and soft drinks by 49kcal. It also seems that many fast food restaurants market the value of a large (e.g., "Super" or "Biggie") size. So for many Americans, larger is better. Unfortunately, a bigger meal also means a heap of calories. A fast food meal comprised of a double cheeseburger, French fries, soft drink, and dessert could easily encompass 2,200 kcal. A person has to run a full marathon in order to burn off all of those calories. (C/17/20 you need this one). Incidentally, the nutrition quality of meals prepared at home are typically better since they are less often fried, have less fat, and are lower on the glycemic index (C/17/21)

The diet of youth today is far from ideal. In the last few decades, fruit and vegetables and milk consumption decreased, while fat and sugary snacks intake increased. In 2001, data on school children revealed that nearly 80% did not consume the recommended servings of fruit, vegetable, dairy, or fiber (Grunbaum see C/17/20). Data from the 2005 Youth Risk Behavior Surveillance System (Center for Disease Control, 2006) revealed that within seven days preceding the national survey, only 20.1% of youth (in grades ninth through twelfth) had eaten five or more than the recommended servings of fruit and vegetables per day. According to Health People 2010 (U.S. Department of Health & Human Services, 2006b), only 3% of Americans eat the recommended three daily servings of vegetables with at least a third or more of the servings being dark green or orange (49% eat three more daily servings of vegetables, while 8% eat at least a third or more of servings that are dark green or orange). Interestingly, research finds that children's fruit and vegetable consumption decreases as they get older. Lytle and his colleagues (2000) found that fruit consumption decreased nearly 40% from the time children were in third grade to the time they were in eighth grade. Their vegetable consumption decreased by 25% during the same time period.

The 2005 Youth Risk Behavior Surveillance System also found that only 16.2% of youth drank more than three glasses of milk per day. Others have noted that more and more youth are replacing milk with soft drinks (Neumark-Sztainer, Story, Resnick, & Blum, 1997; Lytle, 2002). In like manner, data on beverage consumption can lead one to surmise that soft drinks are a staple beverage among youth. From 1989 to 1995, the percentage of soft drink consumption among adolescent males jumped nearly 65%. Nearly a quarter of adolescents drink more than 26 ounces of soda daily, and about 65% of girls and 74% of boys consume soft drinks daily, which constitutes the leading source of added sugar in their diet exceeding the USDA daily recommended sugar consumption (Human Ecology, 2003). Just as potentially damaging are juice drinks that are popular among youngsters. Often parents buy them because they are convenient (a straw even accompanies the box that stacks easily in a kitchen cabinet), and many mistakenly believe that orange, grape, or apple juice drinks are good for their children. However, such drinks can be significant sources of sugar, and if parents substitute actual fruit for juice drinks, children lose out on fiber and other natural nutrients.

Lastly, fat intake concerns many health experts because its consumption in ample doses has been associated with obesity and an increased risk of coronary heart disease. As of 2005, about two out of three persons consumed more than 30% of calories from total fat (U.S. Department of Health & Human Services, 2006b). In other words, a good portion of Americans ate foods that were high in total fat. Unsurprisingly, many youth today consume excess amounts of foods that are high in total fat. Covington and her colleagues (2001) found that nearly 70% of children exceeded the USDA recommended daily allowance of total and saturated fats. Much of this consumption could stem from meals eaten out since researchers have found that children consume high amounts of total and saturated fats when they eat an evening meal away from home (Gonzales, Marshall, Heimendinger, Crane, & Neal, 2002).

Parenting Behaviors and Family Dynamics

Family environment shapes the eating habits of children and youth. Granted, children progressively develop their own food preferences, but during the formative years of their lives they adapt to their familial surroundings and eat what is presented to them – generally their parents' (or caregivers') food preferences. Parents, by way of their own eating habits and attitudes toward food consumption, are direct models for children. They set the norm for food consumption, and early on children learn and develop food preferences, eating habits, and attitudes toward their own intake, especially when certain eating behaviors are encouraged (e.g., snacking while watching TV).

Research has found that the risk of persistent obesity in youth is increased when one or both parents are obese. Children whose parents are obese are at a greater risk of becoming obese than children with one or no obese parents. Myers and Vargas (2000) have pointed out:

- if both parents are obese, there is a 70% chance their children will be obese;
- if one parent is obese, there is an approximate 50% likelihood of obesity in the children; and
- if neither parent is obese, there is only a 10% chance their children will be obese. (e2)

In their exploratory study of 150 children, Agras and his colleagues (2004) found that 64% of children who had overweight parents became overweight themselves, compared to 16% of children whose parents were of normal-weight parents. And, data on 8,494 low-income children, revealed that nearly a quarter of all children born to obese mothers were already obese by the age of four, and obese four year-olds who had obese mothers were three times more likely to continue being obese in childhood (Whitaker, 2004).

Some have argued that parental behaviors directly perpetuate weight gain in children. Researchers have found that mothers of obese children tend to serve them larger portions of food than they do their non-obese children (Waxman & Skunkard, 1980). Others have noted that mothers who reported a greater degree of control over their child's food consumption had children who were less able to internally regulate their intake. In turn, such children had higher body fat (Hood, et al., 2000). And, although television viewing was discussed in a prior section, it is appropriate to interject here that families who eat one or more meals while watching TV eat more red meats, salty foods, soft drinks, and less-nutrient snacks (Coon et al., 2001).

Parents also influence their children's physical activity habits, which in a circuitous way affects their weight status. Quite often children are expected to exercise regularly, yet fewer than half of American children have parents who engage in physical exercise daily (emedicine, 2005). Research has shown that children who watch a lot of TV live in households of adult TV watchers, and children who are sedentary tend to have sedentary parents (Strauss & Knight, 1999; Whitaker et al., 1997).

Another point to address is the issue of parental perception of their children's weight status. Parents rarely recognize when their children are overweight or obese. In a study of low-income New York children whose ages ranged from one to five, only 3% of the parents of children who had a BMI between the 85th and 95th percentile perceived their child as "slightly overweight," and none mentioned that their child was "overweight." For the children whose BMI was greater than the 95th percentile, again only 3% said that their child was "overweight," and 25% rated their child as "slightly overweight." The researchers underscored that the highest prevalence of obesity was among the Hispanic youth, yet Hispanic parents were least likely to recognize overweight or obesity in their children (Tucker, 2000). The data also revealed that mothers of overweight children are not concerned about their child's weight status until they notice that their children are teased or cannot participate in common physical activities. The results of a study on low-income Cincinatti preschool children revealed similar results, but indicated that the mothers believed their children were biologically predisposed to be overweight and they could not affect their weight status (Jain, et al., 2001).

Socioeconomic Status

The last behavioral risk factor associated with childhood obesity is socioeconomic status. Obesity *is* a problem among low-income populations, which strongly suggests that socioeconomic background plays a major role in weight status. For the most part, youth from a higher socioeconomic status are at decreased risk of overweight and obesity. These youth consume more fruit and vegetables than their counterparts from lower socioeconomic status, and they tend to eat 10% or less of foods from saturated fat (Neumark-Sztainer, Story, Hannan, Croll, 2002). Similar findings suggest that adults with higher educational attainment and higher socioeconomic status are also at lower risk for obesity (Wardle, Walfer, & Jarvis, 2002).

Low-income households, on the other hand, are at a higher risk for overweight and obesity. In their study, Goodman, Slap, and Huang (2003) found that lower family income accounted for 32% of obesity among their sample of 15,112 adolescents. Others have also noted that there is a greater prevalence of overweight among youth from lower income families than their peers from higher income families (Troiano & Flegal, 1998). What is particularly worrisome is that the number of American youth living in poverty is climbing. Goodman and her colleagues explain:

> Almost two thirds of adolescents live in homes without a college-education parent, and almost half live in households with incomes below 2.5 times the federal poverty thresholds. Additionally, socioeconomic status inequality is increasing in the United States, which suggests that exposure to lower socioeconomic among teenagers will increase in coming years. (p.5).

Data shows that youth from low-income families are more likely to:
- Consume foods that are high in total and saturated fat, and less likely to eat fruit and vegetables (American Academy of Pediatrics, 2003)
- Eat more sweets and high fat bakery products and sugary and salty snacks (Aranceta, Perez-Rodrigo, Ribas, & Serra-Majem, 2003);
- Watch more TV (Bowman & Harris, 2003); and
- Restrict their children from physical activity and confine them to the indoors (Adams & Benson, 1991).

These elements should surprise few. After all, impoverished families do not have the wherewithal to buy better, healthier foods. Fruits and vegetables, to name a few, tend to be expensive. For instance, during the winter season a Texas chain grocer prices a bag of microwavable broccoli at $2.49 (12 oz.). A parent who is financially struggling could buy that broccoli, or could instead buy a loaf of generic bread (for $.59), wieners ($.62/package), and mustard ($.80/8 oz.) and make hotdogs for three children for less than the price of the broccoli. For their dessert, the same parent could purchase a container of strawberries for $2.99 (one pound). However, a packet of 12 "fun size" Peter Paul candies sells for $.99. The latter satisfies the sweet tooth yet is a fraction of the cost.

One University of California study showed that when low-income families were in financial straits, the consumption of healthier foods declined, while the consumption of cheaper, less nutrient items remained stable (Crawford et al., 2004). Hence, the nutrient inferior foods make sense when finances are tight especially when the parents lack the health knowledge to fully understand the untoward consequences of consistently feeding their children fried foods, sweets, and carbonated beverages. To aggravate matters, some health experts point out that low-income parents often have to work long hours just to make ends meet, which affects their children in two ways:

- Parents may favor and feed their children foods that are easy to prepare, which tend to be high in fat and sodium (Gable & Lutz, 2000); and
- Parents may lack the time to monitor their children's consumption or make meals that can be eaten as a family, and absence of family meals is linked with lower fruit and vegetable intake and higher consumption of fried foods and soft drinks (American Academy of Pediatrics, 2003). One study found that children who lived in a female-headed household watched more TV and had more fat intake than their counterparts who lived with two parents (Bowman & Harris, 2003).

Lastly, because low-income families do not have the luxury to discriminate where they live, many end up in neighborhoods where: fast-food restaurants are more prevalent and offer large tempting valuable meals; small local grocers offer fewer healthier foods; their children are restricted from playing outside because it is unsafe for them (Unger et al, 2004). Many people would say that this is *the* equation for childhood obesity – confined to their homes, watching considerable amounts of TV instead of playing outside, and consuming cheaper, nutrient inferior food.

BASED ON THE RISK FACTORS HOW IS CHILDHOOD OBESITY TREATED?

Health experts recognize the importance of treating childhood obesity; such efforts incontestably avert the onset of medical problems that are closely associated with obesity (Hass et al., 2003). Yet surprisingly, treatment is provided for less than 20% of obese children (Nemet, et al., 2005) and often they are costly with insurance companies reimbursing poorly for weight management programs

(Tershakovec, Watson, Wenner, & Marx, 1999). To complicate matters, childhood obesity is very difficult to treat because prevention and intervention quite often rests at the hands of parents. Of course, treating childhood obesity is the collective responsibility of the individual, family, school, community, food giants, media, and government, but parents have considerable control over their children's health. Some parents may heed the overweight warning and monitor their children's weight, but far more parents may not be willing, or have the time or the resources to learn about nutrition, exercise, behavior modification, and the timing of prevention (Covington et al., 2001). Judging from a prior discussion on parental behaviors, some parents may not even know or believe that their child is overweight or obese and may not duly pursue weight intervention for their child. And, if they do recognize that their child is overweight or obese, they may not know that excess weight is a health issue or may not want to address it assuming that it may cause undue emotional damage.

Treatment of obesity is essential in childhood because it is easier to prevent and treat overweight and obesity in childhood than it is in adulthood (most health experts agree that adults rarely obtain sustained weight loss (Hass et al., 2003)). Reducing the risk of childhood obesity is generally treated by way of health promotion, which encompasses learning about increasing physical activity and altering consumption behaviors – i.e., boost the intake of nutrient-rich foods and scale down on meals, snacks, and beverages that are high in fat, sugar, and sodium. Obesity programs rarely employ weight loss as a goal because a calorie-restricted diet can interrupt growth and development (McArthur, Anguiano, & Gross, 2004). Instead, such programs seek to slow or halt weight gain so that children, in due course (generally months and years), can grow into the optimal body weight (Summerfield, 1990). It is estimated that children need about a year and a half of weight management to attain their ideal weight for every 20% in poundage they have above their average weight (Dietz, 1983). The programs also want to stress upon parents and youth that excess weight is a health issue because often youth relate weight to performance and appearance, but not to health (Food Insight, 2002). A popular newsletter on food and nutrition writes, "Kids are not sure what 'being fit' means and don't sustain interest in concepts like 'nutrition,' 'physical activity,' or 'health eating.' To kids, 'healthy' brings to mind somewhat negative images of being required to eat fruit and vegetables or being deprived of their favorite food. Being healthy equals 'rules'" (Food Insight, 2002, p.e2)

Treatment programs generally want children and adolescents to break the cycle of weight gain. To that end, children are expected to eat a sensible diet and exercise regularly. Iannelli (2007) recommends that treatment encompass:

- Behavior Modification – Here children learn: to limit the amount of television they watch; eat three healthy well-balanced meals with two healthy snacks (e.g., raw fruit or vegetables); drink four to six glasses of water daily, preferably before meals, and limit other drinks to diet sodas and low fat milk; keep a journal of food and beverage consumption; eat at the dining table away from the TV; and avoid fast food.

- Exercise – Here children learn to: exercise for 20-30 minutes for three to four times each week (e.g., walk, jog, swim, bike and so forth); engage in an extracurricular school sports; and walk/bike instead of drive to short distances

Iannelli also advises that youth avoid strict diets that are based on fasting, liquids, or fads, and that the whole family must involve themselves in the intervention, not just a singled-out child. Epstein et al. (1990, 1994) has found that family-centered, multidisciplinary behavior-based programs are effective with as many as 30% of participants at normal weight 10years later. Others add that treatment programs must consider the significance that race and ethnicity have on weight status suggesting that treatment programs address the unique norms of various cultures in terms of body shape perception, eating patterns unique to that culture, and support networks (Neumark-Sztainer, et al., 2002).

A persistent theme in the literature is what is coined obesity knowledge, which is knowing about the direct repercussions of diet, health, and exercise on the body, mind, and spirit. Essentially, health-promotion programs seek to raise the understanding of nutrition and exercise so that individuals can protect themselves from weight gain. As cited earlier, studies repeatedly find that persons from lower socioeconomic status, ethnic backgrounds (particularly Latinos and African Americans), and less formal education have incorrect beliefs about health, which might explain why the prevalence of obesity is higher among them. Thus, some treatments aim to specifically increase parents' nutritional knowledge to alter their attitudes about and behavior toward how they feed their children. This type of parental knowledge influences how parents feed their children (Horodynski, Hoerr, & Coleman, 2004). Some have noted that when mothers' nutritional knowledge increases, they feed their children foods that are lower in fat and higher in fiber (Calovito, Guthrie, Hertzler, Webb, 1996), and others have found that parents can increase their children's acceptance and consumption of healthy foods (Lederman, Akabas, & Moore, 2004).

In the last few years, bariatric surgery has become a common operative procedure for obese adults. Although it is costly – about $25,000—with some insurance companies covering the costs, the surgery has become an alternative treatment for obese adolescents (Freudenheim, 2003). In 2004, the American Academy of Pediatrics devoted a journal issue to the topic of bariatric surgery for youth and underscored that this type of surgery is reserved for severely overweight adolescents. Inge et al. (2004) emphasize:

> For severely overweight adolescents who have failed organized attempts to lose weight and/or to maintain weight loss through conventional nonoperative approaches and who have serious or life-threatening conditions, bariatric surgery may provide the only practical alternative for achieving a healthy weight and for escaping the devastating physical and psychological effects of obesity. (p. 218)

Adolescents who qualify for the surgery have to be severely obese with a BMI greater than or equal to 40 when comorbid conditions exist, and greater than or equal to 50 when there are no comorbid conditions. Medical professionals insist that the surgery be the last resort. Potential candidates should have first justifiably failed organized and credible weight management (conducted by a primary care provider and multidisciplinary team) after more than six months; underwent an exhaustive physical and psychological evaluation; and have medically-based data to support that the surgery will improve and prolong their life. See Table 11 for a list of criteria for bariatric surgery for adolescents.

Table 11. Criteria for bariatric surgery[iv]

Adolescents being considered for bariatric surgery should:
• Have failed more than six months of organized attempts at weight management, as determined by their primary care provider
• Have attained or nearly attained physiologic maturity
• Be very severely obese (BMI >= 40) with serious obesity-related comorbidities or have a BMI of >=50 with less severe comorbidities
• Demonstrate commitment to comprehensive medical and psychological evaluations both before and after surgery
• Agree to avoid pregnancy for at least one year postoperatively
• Be capable of and willing to adhere to nutritional guidelines postoperatively
• Provide informed assent to surgical treatment
• Demonstrate decisional capacity
• Have a supportive family environment

CONCLUSION

The increasing prevalence of childhood obesity is caused by varying factors. While some children gain weight because of non-behavioral factors like genetics or medical conditions, health experts agree that the behavioral factors in the contemporary lifestyle play a major role in the obesity development. Much of the childhood obesity blame rests on children's eating habits and physical inactivity. Children today have higher caloric intake and they lead far more inactive lives compared to generations past. The popularity of TV, the Internet/computers, and video games has called children in away from the more physical activities, and they have fewer opportunities for exercise at school. To complicate matters, there are more palatable foods available to them, yet these are often higher in fat, sugar and sodium. Consuming them adds to the imbalance between energy input (i.e., ample portions of nutrient-inferior foods) and energy output (i.e., sitting with their eyes fixed on screens), which is the very equation for weight gain.

Treatment programs are available for overweight youth, and these tend to promote healthful eating habits and daily exercise by way of behavior modification.

NOTES

[i] Source: Adapted from Moran, R. (1999). Evaluation and treatment of childhood obesity. *American Family Physician, 59(4)*, e12.

[ii] Source: Prader-Willi Syndrome Association. (2006). *The genetics of Prader-Willi Syndrome: An explanation for the rest of us.* Retrieved December 5, 2006, from http://www.pwsausa.org/syndrome/Genetics_of_PWS.htm.

[iii] Source: U.S. Department of Health & Human Services. (2006b). *Healthy people 2010: Nutrition and overweight.* Retrieved February 2, 2007, from
 http://www.healthypeople.gov/Document/pdf/Volume2/19Nutrition.pdf.

[iv] Source: Inge, T., Krebs, N., Garcia, V., Skelton, J., Guice, K., Strauss, R., Albanese, C., Brandt, M., Hammer, L., Harmon, C., Kane, T., Klish, W., Oldham, K., Rudolph, C., Helmrath, M., Donovan, E., & Daniels, S. (2004). Bariatric surgery for severely overweight adolescents: Concerns and recommendations. *Pediatrics, 114(1),* 217-223. Reprinted with permission.

REFERENCES

Adams, P., & Benson, V. (1991). *Current estimates from the National Health Interview Survey, 1990.* (DHHS Publication No. PHS 92-1509). Hyattsville, MD: National Center for Health Statistics.

Agras, W., Hammer, L., McNicholas, F., & Kraemer, H. (2004). Risk factors for childhood overweight: A prospective study from birth to 9.5 years. *Journal of Pediatrics, 145(1),* 20-25.

American Academy of Pediatrics. (2001). Committee on public education: Children, adolescents, and television. *Pediatrics, 107(2),* 423-426.

American Academy of Pediatrics. (2003). Prevention of pediatric overweight and obesity. *Pediatrics, 112(3),* 424-430

American Obesity Association. (2005). *Obesity in minority populations.* Retrieved April 12, 2006, from http://www.obesity.org/subs/fastfacts/Obesity_Minority_Pop.shtml.

American Obesity Association. (2006). *Obesity in youth.* Retrieved December 18, 2006, from http://www.obesity.org/subs/fastfacts/obesity_youth.

American Dietetic Association. (2003). Position of the American Dietetic Association, Society for Nutrition Education, and American School Food Service Association: Nutrition services: An essential component of comprehensive school health programs. *Journal of Nutrition Education & Behavior, 35(2),* e11.

Anderson, R., Crespo, C., Bartlett, S., Cheskin, L., & Pratt. (1998). Relationship of physical activity and television watching with body weight and level of fatness among children: Results from the Third National Health and Nutrition Examination Survey. *JAMA, 279(12),* 938-942.

Aranceta, J., Perez-Rodrigo, C., Ribas, L., & Serra-Majem, L. (2003). Sociodemographic and lifestyle determinants of food patterns in Spanish children and adolescents: The enkid study. *European Journal of Clinical Nutrition, 57(1),* 40-44.

Barlow, S., & Dietz, W. (1998). Obesity evaluation and treatment: Expert committee recommendations. *Pediatrics, 102(3),* e11.

Bauer, L. (2004). The epidemic of childhood obesity: What role do schools play in primary prevention? *Nutrition and Dietetics, 61(3),* 134-135.

Biddle, S., Gorely, T., & Stensel, D. (2004). Health-enhancing physical activity and sedentary behaviour in children and adolescents. *Journal of Sports Sciences, 22(8),* e23.

Bowman, S., & Harris, E. (2003). Food security, dietary choices, and television-viewing status of pre-school-aged children living in single-parent or two-parent households. *Family Economics & Nutrition Review, 15(2),* e8.

Burgeson, C., Wechsler, H., Brener, N., Young, J., & Spain, C. (2001). Physical education and activity: Results from the School Health Policies and Programs Study, 2000. *Journal of School Health, 71(7),* 279-293.

Calavito, E., Guthrie, J., Hertzler, A., & Webb, R. (1996). Relationship of diet-health attitudes and nutrition knowledge of household meal planners to the fat and fiber intakes of meal planners and preschoolers. *Journal of Nutrition Education, 28,* 321-328.

Carmona, R. (2003). *The obesity crises in America.* Retrieved on April 12, 2005, from http://www.surgeongeneral.gov/news/testimony/obesity07162003.htm.

Center for Disease Control. (2005). *Physical activity and health: Adolescents and youth adults.* Retrieved April 12, 2005, from http://www.cdc.gov/nccdphp/sgr/adoles.htm.

Center for Disease Control. (2006). *Youth risk behavior surveillance system – United States, 2005.* Retrieved February 2, 2007, from http://www.cdc.gov/mmwr/PDF/SS/SS5505.pdf.

Clocksin, B., Watson, D., & Ransdell, L. (2002). Understanding youth obesity and media use: Implications for future intervention programs. *Quest, 54(4),* 259-275.

Contento, I., Basch, C., & Zybert, P. (2003). Body image, weight, and food choices of Latina women and their young children. *Journal of Nutrition & Behavior, 35(5),* e21.

Coon, K., Goldberg, J., Rogers, B., & Tucker, K. (2001). Relationship between use of television during meals and children's food consumption patterns. *Pediatrics, 107(1),* e9.

Covington, C., Cybulski, M., Davis, T., Duca, G., Farrell, E., Kasgorgis, M., Kator, C., & Sell, T. (2001). Kids on the move: Preventing obesity among urban children. *AJN, 101(3),* 73-82.

Cowley, G., Pedersen, D., Wingert, P., Weingarten, T., Cooper, A., Gesalman, A., & Gatland, L. (2000). Generation XXL. *Newsweek, 136(1),* p.e4.

Crain, W. (2003). No free ride for toddlers. *New York Times,* September 6, A11.

Crandall, C. (2002). *Polycystic Ovarian Syndrome (PCOS, Stein-Leventhal Syndrome).* Retrieved December 12, 2006, from http://www.medicinenet.com/polycystic_ovary/article.htm.

Crawford, P., Townsend, M., Metz, D., Smith, D., Espinosa-Hall, G., Donohue, S., Olivares, A., & Kaiser, L. (2004). How can Californians be overweight and hungry? *California Agriculture, 58(1),* 12-17.

Crespo, C., & Arbesman, J. (2003). Obesity in the United States. *Physician & Sportsmedicine, 31(1),* e7.

Cushing's-help. (2006). *What is Cushing's.* Retrieved December 11, 2006, from http://www.cushings-help.com/intro.htm.

Dalton, S. (2004). *Our overweight children: What parents, schools, and communities can do to control the fatness epidemic.* Berkeley: CA: University of California Press.

Datar, A., & Sturm, R. (2004). Physical education in elementary school and body mass index: Evidence from the early childhood longitudinal study. *American Journal of Public Health, 94(9),* 1501-1505.

Dennison, B., Erb, T., & Jenkins, P. (2002). Television viewing and television in bedroom associated with overweight risk among low-income preschool children. *Pediatrics, 109(6),* 1028-1035.

Dietz, W. (1983). Childhood obesity: Susceptibility, cause, and management. *Journal of Pediatrics, 103(5),* 676-686.

Dietz, W., & Gortmaker, S. (1985). Do we fatten our children at the television set? Obesity and television viewing in children and adolescents. *Pediatrics, 76(5),* 807-812.

DDC Clinic for Special Needs Children. (2006). *National Cohen Syndrome Support Group.* Retrieved December 5, 2006, from http://www.ddcclinic.org/services_supportgroups.htm.

Drohan, S. (2002). Managing early childhood obesity in the primary care setting: a behavior modification approach. *Pediatric Nursing, 28(6),* 599-610.

Egan, J. (2005). *Can SpongeBob Encourage Healthy Eating?* Retrieved February 11, 2007, from http://www.timeforkids.com/TFK/news/story/0,6260,1139321,00.html.

Emedicine. (2005). *Obesity in children.* Retrieved March 1, 2005 from http://www.emedicinehealth.com/articles/11529-1.asp.

Endocrineinfo.com. (2006). *What is the endocrine system?* Retrieved December 12, 2006, from http://www.endocrine.info/.

Epstein, L., Valoski, A., Wing, R., & McCurley, J. (1990). Ten-year follow-up of behavioral, family-based treatment for obese children. *JAMA, 264(19),* 217-223.

Epstein, L., Valoski, A., Wing, R., & McCurley, J. (1990). Ten-year follow-up of behavioral, family-based treatment for obese children. *JAMA, 264(19)*, 2519-2523.

Ewing, R., Schmid, T., Killingsworth, R., Zlot, A., & Raudenbush, S. (2003). Relationship between urban sprawl and physical activity, obesity, and morbidity. *American Journal of Health Promotion, 18(1)*, 47-57.

Farooqi, I., & O'Rahilly, S. (2000). Recent advances in genetics of severe obesity. *Archives of Diseases in Childhood, 83 (1)*, 31-34.

Flegal, K., Carroll, M., Ogden, C., & Johnson, C. (2002). Prevalence and trends in obesity among US adults, 1999-2000. *JAMA, 288(14)*, 1723-1727.

Food Insight. (2002, July-August). Kidnetic.com: Tap into the energy: Healthful eating and physical activity for kids and parents just a click away. *Food Insight*, pp. 1, 4-5.

Foundation Fighting Blindness. (2006). *Bardet-Biedl syndrome*. Retrieved December 5, 2006, from http://www.blindness.org/visiondisorders/causes.asp?type=27.

Freudenheim, M. (2003). Hospitals pressured by soaring demand for obesity surgery. *New York Times*, retrieved February 10, 2007, from http://query.nytimes.com/gst/fullpage.html?sec=health&res=9F02E5DA1F39F93AA1575BC0A96 59C8B63.

Gable, S., & Lutz, S. (2000). Household, parent, and child contributions to childhood obesity. *Family Relations, 49(3)*, 293-300.

Gonzales, E., Marshall, J., Heimendinger, J., Crane, L., & Neal, W. (2002). Home and eating environments are associated with saturated fat intake in children in rural West Virginia. *Journal of the American Dietetic Association, 102(5)*, 657-663.

Gortmaker, S., Dietz, W., & Cheung, L. (1990). Inactivity, diet and the fattening of America. *Journal of the American Dietetic Association, 90(11)*, 1247-1255.

Gortmaker, S., Must, A., Sobol, A., Peterson, K., Colditz, G., & Dietz, W. (1996). Television viewing as a cause of increasing obesity among children in the United States, 1986-1990. *Archives of Pediatric & Adolescent Medicine, 150(4)*, 356-362.

Grunbaum, J., Kann, L., Kinchen, S., Ross, J., Hawkins, J., Lowry, R., Harris, W., McManus, T., Chyen, D., & Collins, J. (2004). Youth risk behavior surveillance – United States, 2003. *Morbidity and Mortality Weekly Report, 53(2)*, 1-95.

Harrell, J., Gansky, S., Bradley, C., & McMurray, R. (1997). Leisure time activities of elementary school children. *Nursing Research, 46(5)*, 246-253.

Harrell, J., Pearce, P., Markland, E., Wilson, K., Bradley, C., & McMurray, R. (2003). Assessing physical activity in adolescents: Common activities of children in 6th – 8th grades. *Journal of the American Academy of Nurse Practitioners, 15(4)*, 170-177.

Haas, J., Lee, L., Kaplan, C., Sonnenborn, D., Phillips, K., & Liang, S. (2003). The association of race, socioeconomic status, and health insurance status with the prevalence of overweight among children and adolescents. *American Journal of Public Health, 93(12)*, e16.

Horodynski, M., Hoerr, S., & Coleman, G. (2004). Nutrition education aimed at toddlers: A pilot program for rural, low-income families. *Family & Community Health, 27(2)*, 103-113.

Hood, M., Moore, L., Sundarajan-Ramamirti, A., Singer, M., Cupples, L., & Ellison, R. (2000). Parental eating attitudes and the development of obesity in children: The Framingham children's study. *International Journal of Obesity, 24(10)*, 1319-1325.

Human Ecology. (2003, December). Preventing childhood obesity at school, home, and in the community. *Human Ecology*, p. 23.

Iannelli, V. (2007). *Weight management*. Retrieved February 9, 2007, from http://keepkidshealthy.com/adolescent/adolescentproblems/weightmanagement.html.

Inge, T., Krebs, N., Garcia, V., Skelton, J., Guice, K., Strauss, R., Albanese, C., Brandt, M., Hammer, L., Harmon, C., Kane, T., Klish, W., Oldham, K., Rudolph, C., Helmrath, M., Donovan, E., & Daniels, S. (2004). Bariatric surgery for severely overweight adolescents: Concerns and recommendations. *Pediatrics, 114(1)*, 217-223.

Institute of Medicine. (2004a). *Advertising, marketing and the media: Improving messages*. Retrieved March 1, 2006, from http://www.iom.edu/Object.File/Master/22/606/FINALfactsandfigures2.pdf.

Institute of Medicine. (2004b). *Childhood obesity in the United States: Facts and figures*. Retrieved December 6, 2006, from http://www.iom.edu/Object.File/Master/22/609/fact%20sheet%20-%20marketing%20finaBitticks.pdf

Jain, A., Sherman, S., Chamberlin, L., Carter, Y., Powers, S., & Whitaker, R. (2001). Why don't low-income mothers worry about their preschoolers being overweight? *Pediatrics, 107(5)*, e17.

Jordan, A., Hersey, J., McDivitt, J., & Heitzler, C. (2006). Reducing children's television-viewing time: A qualitative study of parents and their children. *Pediatrics, 118(5),*1303-1310.

Kaiser Family Foundation. (2004). *The role of media in childhood obesity*. Menlo Park, CA: Kaiser Family Foundation.

Kimm, S. (1995). The role of dietary fiber in the development and treatment of childhood obesity. *Pediatrics, 96(5)*, e5.

Klesges, R., Shelton, M., & Klesges, L. (1993). Effects on television on metabolic rate: potential implications for childhood obesity. *Pediatrics, 91(2)*, 281-286.

Lavizzo-Mourey, R., & McGinnis, J. (2003). Making the case for active living communities. *American Journal of Public Health, 93(9)*, 1386-1388.

Lederman, S., Akabas, S., & Moore, B. (2004). Editors' overview of the conference on preventing childhood obesity. *Pediatrics, 114(4)*, 1139-1145.

Louie, D., Sanchez, E., Faircloth, S., & Dietz, W. (2003). School-based policies: Nutrition and physical activity. *Journal of Law, Medicine, & Ethics, 31(4)*, 73-75.

Lowry, R., Weschler, H., Galuska, D., Fulton, J., & Kann, L. (2002). Television viewing and its association with overweight, sedentary lifestyle, and insufficient consumption of fruits and vegetables among US high school students: Differences by race, ethnicity, and gender. *Journal of School Health, 72(10)*, e9.

Ludwig, D., & Gortmaker, S. (2004). Programming obesity in childhood. *The Lancet, 364(9430)*, 226-227.

Lynn-Garb, C., & Hoot, J. (2004/5). Weighing in on the issue of childhood obesity. *Childhood Education, 81(2)*, 70-76.

Lytle, L. (2002). Nutritional issues for adolescents. *Journal of the American Dietetic Association, 102(3)*, S8-S12.

Lytle, L., Seifert, S., Greenstein, J., & McGovern, P. (2000). How do children's eating patterns and food choices change over time? Results from a cohort study. *American Journal of Public Health, 41(14)*, 222-228.

Maddock, J. (2004). The relationship between obesity and the prevalence of fast food restaurants: State-level analysis. *American Journal of Health Promotion, 19(2)*, 137-143.

Marr, L. (2004). Soft drinks, childhood overweight, and the role of nutrition educators: Let's base our solutions on reality and sound science. *Society for Nutrition Education, 36(5)*, 258-263.

Mayoclinic.com. (2006a). *Cushing's syndrome*. Retrieved December 11, 2006, from http://www.mayoclinic.com/health/cushings-syndrome/DS00470.

Mayoclinic.com. (2006b). *Hypothyroidism*. Retrieved December 11, 2006, from http://www.mayoclinic.com/health/hypothyroidism/DS00353/DSECTION=2.

Massey-Stokes, M. (2002). Adolescent nutrition. *Clearing House, 75(6)*, e6.

Matheson, D., Killen, J., Wang, Y., Varady, A., & Robinson, T. (2004). Children's food consumption during television viewing. *American Journal of Clinical Nutrition, 79(6)*, 1088-1094.

McArthur, L., Anguiano, R., & Gross, K. (2004). Are household factors putting immigrant Hispanic children at risk of becoming overweight: A community-based study in Eastern North Carolina. *Journal of Community Health, 29(5)*, e14.

Medline Plus. (2006a). *Cushing's syndrome*. Retrieved December 11, 2006, from http://www.nlm.nih.gov/medlineplus/ency/article/000410.htm.

Medline Plus. (2006b). *Hypothyroidism*. Retrieved December 11, 2006, from http://www.nlm.nih.gov/medlineplus/ency/article/000353.htm.

Mokdad, A., Serdula, M., Dietz, W., Bowman, B., Marks, J., & Koplan, J. (2000). The continuing epidemic of obesity in the US. *JAMA, 284(13)*, 1650-1651.

Montague, M. (2003). The physiology of obesity. *The ABNF Journal*, 56-60.

Myers, S., & Vargas, Z. (2000). Parental perceptions of the preschool obese child. *Pediatric Nursing, 26(1)*, e8.

National Association for Sport and Physical Education. (2006). *Shape of the nation report: Status of physical education in the USA*. Oxon Hill, MD: AAHPERD.

National Center for Health Statistics. (2002). *National health and nutrition examination survey: Table 70*. Retrieved April 12, 2005, from http://www.obesity.org/subs/fastfacts/Obesity_Minority_Pop.shtml.

National Center for Health Statistics. (2004). *Obesity still a major problem, new data show.* Retrieved March 22, 2005, from http://www.cdc.gov/nchs/pressroom/04facts/obesity.htm.

National Organization for Rare Disorders. (2006). *Cohen syndrome.* Retrieved December 5, 2006, from http://www.rarediseases.org/search/rdbdetail_abstract.html?disname=Cohen%20Syndrome.

National Center for Health Statistics. (2006). *Prevalence of overweight among children and adolescents: United States, 1999-2000.* Retrieved December 06, 2006, from http://www.cdc.gov/nchs/products/pubs/pubd/hestats/overwght99.htm.

Nemet, D., Barkan, S., Epstein, Y., Friedland, O., Kowan, G., & Eliakim, A. (2005). Short- and long-term beneficial effects of a combined dietary-behavioral-physical activity intervention for the treatment of childhood obesity. *Pediatrics, 115(4),* e6.

Nemours Foundation. (2006). *Endocrine system.* Retrieved December 12, 2006, from http://kidshealth.org/parent/general/body_basics/endocrine.html.

Neumark-Sztainer, D., Story, M., Dixon, L., Resnick, M., & Blum, R. (1996). Correlates of inadequate consumption of dairy products among adolescents. *Journal of Nutrition Education, 29(1),* 12-20.

Neumark-Sztainer, D., Story, M., Hannan, P., & Croll, J. (2002). Overweight status and eating patterns among adolescents: Where do youths stand in comparison with the Healthy People 2010 objectives. *American Journal of Public Health, 92(5),* e8.

Ogden, C., Flegal, K., Carroll, M., & Johnson, C. (2002). Prevalence and trends in overweight among US children and adolescents, 1999-2000. *JAMA, 288(14),* 1728-1732.

Parizkova, J., & Hills, A. (2001). *Childhood obesity: Prevention and treatment.* Washington, DC: CRC Press.

Prader-Willi Syndrome Association. (2006). *Questions and answers on Prader-Willi Syndrome.* Retrieved December 5, 2006, from http://www.pwsausa.org/faq.htm.

Rideout, V., Foerh., U., Roberts, D., & Brodie, M. (1999). *Kids & media@ the new millennium. Kaiser Family Foundation Report.* Menlo Park, CA: Kaiser Family Foundation.

Robbins, L., Andersen, G., & Morandi, L. (2004). What's health got to do with it? *State legislature, 30(6),* e6.

Robinson, T. (1998). Does television cause childhood obesity? *JAMA, 279(12),* 959-960.

Robinson, T. (1999). Reducing children's television viewing to prevent obesity: A randomized controlled trial. *JAMA, 282(16),* 1561-1567

Robinson, T., & Killen, J. (1995). Ethnic and gender difference in the relationships between television viewing and obesity, physical activity, and dietary fat intake. *Journal of Health Education, 26(2),* S91-S96.

Rosenthal, M. (1998). *Polycystic Ovarian Syndrome.* Retrieved December 12, 2006, from http://www.webmd.com/content/article/4/1680_51208.

Saltmarsh, N. (2001, June 25). Low-income mothers judge children's weight using their own criteria. *Health & Medicine Week,* pp.14.

Smith, J. (1999). *Understanding childhood obesity.* Jackson, MS: University Press of Mississippi.

Stanger, J. (1998). *Television in the home 1998: The third annual national survey of parents and children.* Philadelphia, PA: Annenberg Public Policy Center.

Storey, M., Forshee, R., Weaver, A., & Sansalone, W. (2003). Demographic and lifestyle factors associated with body mass index among children and adolescents. *International Journal of Food Sciences and Nutrition, 54(6),* 491-503.

Strauss, R., & Knight, J. (1999). Influence of the home environment on the development of obesity in children. *Pediatrics, 103(6),* e8.

Strock, G., Cottrell, E., Abang, A., Buschbacher, R., & Hannon, T. (2005). Childhood obesity: A simple equation with complex variables. *Journal of Long-Term Effects of Medical Implants, 15(1),* 15-32.

Tershakovec, A., Watson, M., Wenner, W., & Marx, A. (1999). Insurance reimbursement for the treatment of obesity in children. *Journal of Pediatrics, 134(5),* 573-578.

Thompson, C., & Shanley, E. (2004). *Overcoming childhood obesity.* Boulder, CO: Bull Publishing Company.

Troiano, R., & Flegal, K. (1998). Overweight children and adolescents: Description, epidemiology, and demographics. *Pediatrics, 101(3),* 497-501.

Tucker, M. (2000). Obese children often seen as normal by low-income parents. *Family Practice News, 30(17),* 42.

73

Unger, J., Reynolds, K., Shakib, S., Spruijt-Metz, D., Sun, P., & Johnson, C. (2004). Acculturation, physical activity, and fast-food consumption among Asian-American and Hispanic adolescents. *Journal of Community Health, 29(6),* e15.

U.S. Department of Health & Human Services. (2006a). *Healthy people 2010.* Retrieved December 26, 2006, from http://www.healthypeople.gov/Default.htm.

U.S. Department of Health & Human Services. (2006b). *Healthy people 2010: Nutrition and overweight.* Retrieved February 2, 2007, from
http://www.healthypeople.gov/Document/pdf/Volume2/19Nutrition.pdf.

U.S. Department of Health & Human Services. (2006c). *Polycystic Ovarian Syndrome (PCOS).* Retrieved December 12, 2006, from http://www.4woman.gov/faq/pcos.htm.

U.S. Department of Health & Human Services. (2006d). Youth risk behavior surveillance – United States, 2005. *Morbidty and Mortality Weekly Report, 55(22-5),* 1-108.

Wardle, J., Walfer, J., & Jarvis, M. (2002). Sex differences in the association of socioeconomic status with obesity. *American Journal of Public Health, 92(8),* e14.

Weicha, J., Sobol, A., Peterson, K., & Gortmaker, S. (2001). Household television access: Assocations with screen time, reading and homework. *Ambulatory Pediatrics, 1(5),* 244-251.

Wharton, C., & Hampl, J. (2004). Beverage consumption and risk of obesity among Native Americas in Arizona. *Nutrition Reviews, 62(4),* 153-158.

Whitaker, R., Wright, J., Pepe, M., Seidel, K., & Dietz, W. (1997). Predicting obesity in young adulthood from childhood and parental obesity. *The New England Journal of Medicine, 337(13),* 869-873.

Wikipedia. (2006). *Prader-Willi Syndrome.* Retrieved December 5, 2006, from
http://en.wikipedia.org/wiki/Prader-Willi_syndrome.

Yackel, E. (2003). An activity calendar progam for children who are overweight. *Pediatric Nursing, 29(1),* 17-22.

HEALTH PROMOTION AT SCHOOL

If we fail to address the issue of childhood obesity, children and adolescents alike will continue to make poor health choices that lead to chronic diseases and diet-associated health problems. In short, their quality of life will be negatively affected. Former U.S. Surgeon General Richard Carmona (2003) expressed that society cannot afford to tolerate the public's poor health choices adding that the health crises we are in must be addressed so that "our children and grandchildren inherit a legacy of health and wellness from us" (e2). Thus, for the sake of our nation's current and future health, health promotion programs that reach the masses are essential to alter the way we eat and how we expend our energy.

Obesity has become a special area of interest for public health officials. Carmona has identified three priorities for immediate action, one of which includes communication (U.S. Department of Health and Human Services, 2007). The priority states:

The Nation must take an informed, sensitive, approach to communicate with and educate the American people about health issues related to overweight and obesity. Everyone must work together to:

- Change the perception of overweight and obesity at all ages. The primary concern should be one of health and not appearance....
- Educate about obesity across the lifespan
- Provide culturally appropriate education in schools and communities about healthy eating habits and regular physical activity, based on the dietary guidelines for Americans, for people of all ages. Emphasize the consumer's role in making wise food and physical activity choices. (e1)

Among the key words in this priority is "everyone," and everyone, including school personnel, shares the collective responsibility of the obesity epidemic solution. Feeg (2004) points out, "The [childhood obesity] problem cannot be approached with simplistic, singular finger-pointing, and requires a positive and united attack on all levels" (p. 361). To that end, schools play an important role in helping youth learn healthy behaviors that can last a lifetime.

This chapter examines how schools can intervene in this major public health concern known as childhood obesity. A discourse follows with specific attention to the following questions:

- Why should my school institute a health promotion program?
- What can I do at my school and in my classroom?
- How should I approach my students who are overweight or obese?

WHY SHOULD MY SCHOOL INSTITUTE A HEALTH PROMOTION PROGRAM?

Many children today have poor dietary and exercise habits. Fast and other non-nutritious foods and soft drinks are readily available in their lives and they generally prefer them to more nutrient-rich alternatives. Many youth positively associate snacking with sedentary activities, and children are increasingly drawn to more sedentary activities than to physical ones. Schools can lead children and youth away from these and other bad habits and help them make long-lasting favorable changes that establish healthful behaviors (Horodynski, Hoerr, & Coleman, 2004). Schools can systematically target children early and teach them healthy decision-making skills, which is critical because often bad dietary habits and lack of exercise in adulthood are established early in life. Schools can teach children the knowledge associated with weight gain and promote the value of a healthy life to shape their attitudes toward their own health and well being.

Schools are ideal settings for grand-scale health promotion programs because they reach wide audiences. On any given day, schools can reach an impressive number of youth. About 95% of the nation's youth between the ages of five and 17 years-old are enrolled in schools, and they spend more time in classrooms than any other place than home (American Dietetic Association et al., 2003). Schools are such an integral part of their lives because youth spend nearly their first two decades of life in school environments, which means that they can learn initial health information and get continuous reinforcement for making healthy choices. In fact, schools may be the only natural environment where they get correct health knowledge and engage in physical activity.

Youth can certainly receive health promotion information by other means such as from an event at a community center, but it would have to be attractive and convenient enough to draw in the community. And, the amount of persons they could attract would compare poorly to the numbers that schools pull in. Of course, pediatricians or their clinics could deliver the health promotion message, but this might prove costly for parents. Those parents with insurance coverage may remit inexpensive co-pays, but there is still the matter of taking time off of work to make the trip to the doctor. What is to say of families with no insurance and parents who do not have the luxury of taking time away from work? The pediatrician route is somewhat limited given that physicians see about 25 patients a day. Even if pediatricians nationwide devoted entire clinical sessions delivering obesity prevention information, they still could not reach the 56 million (or so) youth that schools do.

Schools have the added advantage of having natural facilities to accommodate sizeable audiences. Because parents are already stakeholders in their children's education, many of them are familiar with teachers and the education system and are actively involved in PTAs. What better setting could there be for parents to participate in learning about the behaviors associated with children's weight control? Not to mention that a school-based health promotion program eliminates the need for parents to transport children to another site. Schools also have the unique feature of the federally supported lunch program and built-in cafeteria services. Many children nationwide (in 2003 about 51% participated in the National School Lunch Program and 13% participated in the School Breakfast Program) consume much of their nutritional needs by way of school-served meals, which makes it convenient to directly improve children's diet. School personnel can discuss nutrition, food choices, and so forth and then guide and positively reinforce children in the breakfast and lunch line.

Schools can also indirectly mold the eating and physical activity of youth through the interactions they have with their peers. Research has shown that familial influences decrease as youth get older. Perez-Rodrigo and Aranceta (2003) elaborate:

> During school age, the social environment of children diversifies and extrafamilial influences progressively become more important references. In this period, children are more independent, start making their own food choices and take personal decisions regarding what they eat. The family is less important for adolescents, while friends, peers and social models are the key influences on their eating practices. (p. S82)

Schools are the very laboratory in which youth can regularly reinforce one another about healthy choices they make now and later in life. Moreover, if schools want, they can create special programs to sustain weight control through a peer support system (likened to the adult commercial version of Weight Watchers or LA Weight Loss, etc.), which can be led by a counselor, nurse or district dietician. Children and their parents who express interest in such a program could meet regularly to check-in with one another, learn healthy practices, and monitor their weight control.

Schools should become involved in the obesity epidemic solution because it is axiomatic that children who are healthy – mentally and physically fit – are more likely to learn and perform well in school than children who are not. Studies have found a direct correlation between good nutrition and fitness and improved academic performance (Coles, 2004). The American Dietetic Association et al.(2003) writes:

> One of the strongest justifications for nutrition programs and services in schools is the effect on students' cognitive performance and their educational achievement. Good nutrition is linked to learning readiness and academic achievement, decreased discipline problems, and decreased emotional problems. (p. e3)

Research also suggests that even when physical education time is increased and allocated from instructional time, academic achievement still increases (Human

Ecology, 2003). Ergo, students do better when they eat better, and this applies to their motor development as well. One study of leisure behavior among 668 children found that those who were more physically active had better gross motor development (Graf, et al., 2004).

Health experts have found that once obesity develops it is difficult to treat suggesting that prevention is easier than treatment (Davis, Davis, Northington, Moll, & Kolar, 2002). Others have noted that children are vulnerable to weight gain in early childhood and in adolescence (Brownlee, Martens, McDowell, & Sieger, 2002), which may be attributed to the idea that they develop poor, unwavering health habits early in their lives making it increasingly difficult to alter as they get older. For this reason, schools become important places for health promotion programs because early prevention efforts can hinder youth from fostering such patterns. To borrow words from an old adage, it is best to enlighten youth before they are fixed in their ways. School-based efforts that start in the primary grades can get to them before eating poor-nutrient foods are a practice and sedentary activities are a favorite pastime.

School-based obesity prevention programs are also purposeful because some have been proven to be more effective than those conducted outside schools (Fren et al., 2003). Barlow, Trowbridge, Klish, and Dietz (2002) explain that school-based programs focused on improved eating and activity behavior can lead to sustained weight loss and that intervention in childhood may be a particularly effective means to prevent obesity and reduce excess weight. Veugulers and Fitzgerald (2005) assert that school-based programs work. They studied the BMI, dietary intake, and physical activities of 5,200 fifth grade students and discovered that students who participated in a school-based healthy eating program had lower rates of overweight and obesity, healthier diets, and were more frequently engaged in physical activity than students in schools without such nutrition-focused programs. Their data also revealed that having an alternative healthy menu at school without health/nutrition instruction is insufficient in helping students maintain a healthy body weight. The authors concluded that students who were in schools with health programs consistent with the Centers for Disease Control recommendations for school-based healthy eating programs were less likely to be overweight and obese.

A study conducted by a research team from the University of North Carolina evaluated the total cholesterol and LDL (bad cholesterol) levels of 600 11- to 14-years-olds prior to their participation in a school-based obesity reduction program. The children were divided into four groups: those that would receive instruction about nutrition, smoking, fitness, and cardiovascular (twice/week); those that would participate in a physical activity program for 20 to 30 minutes (thrice/week); those that would participate in both programs; and those that were the control group. At the end of the study, the students who were involved in both programs had the greatest reduction in total cholesterol (Davis, Davis, Northington, Moll, & Kolar, 2002). On the surface this might not seem like such great news because the youth did not report drastic weight loss; however, the study confirmed that a school-based program can significantly reduce one of the major risks associated with cardiovascular disease.

Robert G. McMurray, professor of exercise and nutrition at University of North Carolina, also espouses that school-based programs work, but adds that a vigorous exercise program will reduce the risk that youth will develop serious chronic diseases (McMurray, Harrell, Bangdiwala, Bradley, Deng, & Levine, 2002). McMurray and his associates found that by boosting the amount of exercise middle school children received, they were able to control the students' body fat and lower their blood pressure. Similar studies have noted that students' physical activity level increases when programs are focused on improving their knowledge and attitudes toward physical activity (Stone, McKenzie, Welk, & Booth, 1998). In a study that examined the effect of physical education instruction time on the BMI of 9,751 kindergarteners, Datar and Sturm (2004) determined that an extra hour of physical education a week reduced BMI among girls who were overweight or at risk of overweight. The authors concluded, "On the basis of our estimates, expanding existing PE instruction time nationwide so that every kindergartener gets at least 5 hours of PE instruction per week (close to the recommended levels) could decrease the prevalence of overweight among girls by 4.2 percentage points (43%) and the prevalence of children who are at risk for overweight by 9.2 percentage points (60%)" (p.1504). It is important to note that while research suggest that some school-based programs are effective, other programs, especially those described in the seminal work of Fowler-Brown and Kahwati (2004) and Baranowski et al. (2002), are not. Thorpe et al. (2004) adds that the number of school-based interventions is limited and often the programs are modestly successful. The authors do not elaborate why some programs are ill-fated, but it can be inferred that those programs were not extensive, ongoing, and subject to restricted conditions.

Schools should institute obesity reduction/health promotion programs because youth deserve to take an active role in their own physical health and well-being. Simply put, children need help in developing obesity knowledge. As discussed in Chapter Three, youth are cognitively vulnerable (especially the youngsters) to the messages they see and hear from media. Many of them believe that just because fast foods and other nutrient-inferior snacks exist and are available to them, they must be good for them especially when there are many clever jingles promoting so many food products. Obesity knowledge can help them distinguish what is good and what is good for them. It can be particularly beneficial to adolescents who believe that dieting is an effective means for weight control. Many teens assume that dieting is acceptable because adult-based diets are pervasive in our society. Teens may read about fad diets in popular tabloids, watch reality shows that transform heavier persons into thinner ones by way of quick weight loss, see commercials for weight control centers or pills that help lose weight and assume that dieting is good for them, when in fact it is not. Dieting, especially in the cycle of chronic weight gain and loss, threatens the physical body of an adolescent and has been linked to coronary heart disease and other deadly eating disorders

(Covington et al., 2001). This is particularly frightening considering that as many as half of female adolescents report they diet to lose weight.

Finally, a leading reason for instituting a school health promotion program in your school is because youth seem to want them. Various researchers have noted that adolescents have expressed interest in participating in obesity education programs. McArthur, Pena, and Holbert (2001), for instance, found that Latin American youth from high and low income families were receptive to obesity education opportunities, and that others, namely Neumark-Sztainer and Story (1997), reported similar findings with overweight adolescents wanting to participate in a school-based weight management program. Also, in their study of ninth grade students, James, Reinzo, and Frazee (1997) discovered that the teens wanted to watch videos featuring other adolescents dealing with nutrition, fitness, weight control, and so forth. Based on findings such as these, it is reasonable to infer that youth want to be healthy and fit, and this can be accomplished through school-based programs that can encourage and help them make healthier choices in their lives.

WHAT CAN I DO AT MY SCHOOL AND IN MY CLASSROOM?

Schools can help reverse the childhood obesity trend through efforts made in and outside of the classroom. Through a school-based comprehensive health and physical education program, youth can better understand their eating and physical activity patterns and develop decision-making skills that lead to healthful dietary and exercise behaviors. You and your colleagues can impart those skills and provide students with the support they need to maintain a healthy lifestyle. In fact, your school is mandated to.

According to federal law PL 108-265, Child Nutrition and Women, Infant, and Children (WIC) reauthorization Act of 2004 (an amendment to the National School Lunch Act), your school district has to have a plan, called the Wellness Policy, in effect that outlines actions to improve student health and help reduce childhood obesity. Hardy (2004) adds, "The policy asks schools to promote exercise and healthier eating and to incorporate nutrition education into physical education classes, health classes, and after-school programs, including athletics" (p.8). Table 12 lists some of the most frequently asked questions regarding the number of ways that your school can meet the wellness policy requirements. Namely, endeavors in nutrition education, physical education, and meals and foods served during the school day can induce healthy changes.

Nutrition Education

The primary purpose of nutrition education is to teach students to adopt a daily balanced diet. School personnel can kick-start nutrition-related skills by way of fun, interactive developmentally appropriate and culturally relevant practices (Massey-Stokes, 2002). Help develop or adopt innovative programs that teach and support students to pass on the nutritionally empty, calorie-laden foods that are

Table 12. FAQ about Wellness Policy requirements[i]

---

1. What is the Local Wellness Policy? The Local Wellness Policy requirement is established by *Section 204 of the Public Law 108-265*, the Child Nutrition and WIC Reauthorization Act of 2004. It requires each local education agency (LEA) or school district participating in the National School Lunch Program and/or School Breakfast Program to develop a local wellness policy that promotes the health of students and addresses the growing problem of childhood obesity.

2. Why does a school district need a Local Wellness Policy? The Local Wellness Policy is important because it: reaches beyond USDA-funded meal programs to influence children's health; acknowledges local community responsibility to support or build on government efforts; provides an opportunity for school districts to create an environment conducive to healthy lifestyle choices; and, recognizes the critical role of schools in curbing the epidemic of childhood overweight and obesity.

3. What does the policy require from school districts? A local wellness policy for schools shall, at a minimum: include goals for nutrition education, physical activity and other school- based activities that are designed to promote student wellness in a manner that the local educational agency determines is appropriate; include nutrition guidelines selected by the local educational agency for all foods available on each school campus under the local educational agency during the school day with the objectives of promoting student health and reducing childhood obesity; provide an assurance that guidelines for reimbursable school meals shall not be less restrictive than regulations and guidance issued by the Secretary of Agriculture pursuant to subsections (a) and (b) of section 10 of the Child Nutrition Act (42 U.S.C. 1779) and section 9(f)(1) and 17(a) of the Richard B Russell National School Lunch Act (42 U.S.C. 1758(f)(1), 1766(a)0, as those regulations and guidance apply to schools; establish a plan for measuring implementation of the local wellness policy, including designation of 1 or more persons within the local educational agency or at each school, as appropriate, charged with operational responsibility for ensuring that the school meets the local wellness policy; and involve parents, students, and representatives of the school food authority, the school board, school administrators, and the public in the development of the school wellness policy.

4. Who needs to be involved? A team of community members should be involved in the development of each local wellness policy. Parents, students, and representatives of the school food authority, the school board, school administrators, and the public should be a part of the process. For more information, visit the *Identifying a Policy Development Team.*

5. What are the deadlines? Districts must establish local wellness policies by the beginning of School Year 2006-2007, but local wellness policies are an ongoing project. They should be continuously implemented, evaluated, and updated.

6. Where can I get more information and technical support? USDA has developed wellness web-resources, as a part of the Team Nutrition website. The Local Wellness Policy web-pages are a clearinghouse for information, with web pages on policy requirements, sample policy language, examples of existing State and district policies in various wellness topics, the local process (i.e. how to create and implement a local wellness policy), reference materials, and links to more resources.

7. Are Residential Child Care Institutions (RCCIs) expected to have a wellness policy, in compliance with the requirement in Section 204 of the CN and WIC Reauthorization Act? Yes, they are. FNS is aware that the people involved in developing the wellness policy might be different than those specified in the law and/or used by a school district. For example, in certain RCCIs, it may be impossible to include a parent with the list of people specified in the law for development of a local wellness policy. Because of the responsibility the RCCI has in providing nutrition and physical activity to children in residence, FNS believes it is important for each RCCI to address wellness policies that will affect the health and development of its residents. It is therefore expected that the RCCI will individualize the wellness policy to meet the unique needs of its institution.

8. Are all schools within an LEA that participate in our school meals programs (including the National School Lunch Program, School Breakfast Program and Special Milk Program), bound by the LEA wellness policy, even if a school within the LEA does not participate in any of the programs? No. Schools within the LEA that do not participate in any of the school meals programs are not legally required to be bound by the LEA's local wellness policies. However, for consistency, FNS feels that most LEAs will require schools to follow the district policy.

9. Does the wellness policy requirement apply to private schools, including religious private schools, and charter schools? Yes. Any school that participates in a program authorized under the National School Lunch Act or the Child Nutrition Act must develop a local wellness policy as specified in the Section 204 of the Public Law 108-265, the Child Nutrition and WIC Reauthorization Act of 2004.

10. Do private schools develop their own wellness policy or must they follow the local school district's wellness policy? Private schools or charter schools may develop their own wellness policy or, as in the case of parochial schools, the governing board could develop one for all their schools. A private school could also adopt the wellness policy of the local educational agency.

11. Are schools, including private schools that participate in only the Special Milk Program required to develop a wellness policy? Yes. Schools that participate in the SMP must have a wellness policy. Considering the special circumstances for schools that only participated in the Special Milk Program, these schools may want to consider adopting a wellness policy developed by a local educational agency.

Questions are frequently updated. For the latest information, log on to:
http://teamnutrition.usda.gov/Healthy/wellnesspolicy.html

familiar, tempting, and appetizing like pizza, French fries, and snack cakes – foods that can leave them deceptively satisfied, and instead select the nutritional items, like baked chicken, salad and fruit cups that are filling yet good for them. Covington and her colleagues (2001) explain:

> A snack consisting of a sandwich made with natural peanut butter, all-fruit preserves, and whole-wheat bread; a banana; and low-fat milk, 100% juice enriched with calcium, or water represents approximately the same number of calories as a snack consisting of a cola, a candy bar, and a bag of chips (around 600 to 700 calories). Yet the sandwich snack provides needed nutrients: protein, carbohydrates, unsaturated vegetable fat, and vitamins and minerals. The junk-food snack is high in carbohydrates but deficient in protein, vitamins A, C, and E and folate. (p. 79)

Some of the nutrition skills-based objectives to consider include:

1) Learn about the nutritional value of foods.   Through nutrition education, students can learn the fundamentals of calories, fat, carbohydrates, cholesterol, protein, sodium, and so forth, and how much they should consume in a given day according to their age, weight and height, and gender. Moreover, they can be taught to limit their consumption of trans fats, cholesterol, added sugars, and salt.

The Dietary Guidelines for Americans (U.S. Department of Health and Human Services, 2005) is one of the best blueprints for healthy eating and a great initial resource to direct young people to choose the right nutritional diet. The *Dietary Guidelines* were first released in 1980 and have since been revised every five years to reflect the latest scientific research and information provided by the Dietary Guidelines Advisory Committee (appointed jointly by the U.S. Department of Health and Human Services and the U.S. Department of Agriculture). The most current edition is the 2005 issue with key recommendations subsumed under nine rubrics: adequate nutrients within calorie needs; weight management; physical activity; food groups to encourage; fats, carbohydrates; sodium and potassium; alcoholic beverages; and food safety. While nutrition education should be exhaustive with sequential lessons specific to recommended practices, discussed here are a few items to address.

Calories. While the term calorie is seemingly mentioned in most food commercials and diet products, not all youth will know what a calorie is and how it is derived. At the introductory nutrition education phase, youth can learn that calories in foods are measured with a device known as a calorimeter that burns food, and the amount of heat that is produced is measured. It takes one calorie to raise the temperature of one gram of water by one degree Celsius. Youth can also learn that a calorie is a source of energy for normal body functioning, and that it is *the* metaphoric fuel that keeps the body going (Kirschmann & Nutrition Search, Inc., 2007).

Teach youth that the body burns a certain number of calories to run the body; the rest is expended by additional physical activities and exercise. The body converts the excess into glycogen, which is stored all over the body as fat (Kirschmann & Nutrition Search, Inc., 2007). A high consumption of calories can consequently lead to increased levels of body fat. The daily calorie requirements range from 1,600 to 2,800 depending on a person's size, gender, age, genetic makeup, and physical activity level. According to Bauer (2005), 2,200 calories is about right for most children and teenage girls, whereas teenage boys tend to need about 2,800 calories. Individual daily calorie quotas, however, can be determined at MyPyramid.gov (use the MyPyramid Plan button to retrieve an individualized quota after entering specific age, gender, weight, height, and level of physical activity information).

It is particularly important to underscore that students should choose a diet that has enough calories for their unique, growing bodies and that they should never restrict their calorie intake because they believe they are too heavy (Ward, 2005). In this vain, stress that they should monitor what and how much they eat but not to the point of counting every calorie (Bauer).

Fats. Fats should be addressed in great length primarily because fad diets over the last few decades have promoted them as the sure path to obesity. While fats have gotten a bad rap over the last few years, fats are vital to good health. They are a natural part of a diet that support the absorption of fat-soluble vitamins A, D, E, and K, aid in membrane building, and regulate a number of biological functions (Dietary Guidelines for Americans, 2005). Additionally, fats affect the taste (generally for the better), texture, and appearance of foods, and can leave a person feeling full and satisfied after a meal (Montague, 2003). Bauer (2005) adds:

- Children need fat to grow properly;
- Fat supplies essential fatty acids that your body can't make and must therefore get from foods;
- Fat helps promote healthy skin and hair;
- Fat provides a layer of insulation just beneath the skin; and
- Fat surrounds your vital organs for protection and support. (p.36)

But high consumption of saturated and trans fats (and cholesterol) increase the risk of coronary heart disease.

There are four different kinds of fats: saturated, polyunsaturated, monounsaturated, and trans fat. Saturated fat can be harmful to your health. The body produces all of the saturated fat it needs, the excess saturated fat, which we consume from dairy products, the animal fats in meats, coconut oil and so forth, increases the risk of a heart condition known as Atherosclerosis (the narrowing or blocking of the arteries) that leads to heart attacks and strokes. Scientific research suggests that unsaturated fat is good fat because it supplies fatty acids and helps stabilize blood cholesterol levels to a normal level (Ward, 2005). Polyunsaturated and monounsaturated are endorsed as heart healthy and can be found in a range of foods like: soybean oil, olive oil, avocados, and nuts. Trans fat made national headlines in late 2006 when the New York City Department of Health and Mental

Hygiene banned restaurants from frying with oils that contain trans fats. Trans fat is particularly destructive because it raises the body's cholesterol. Trans fat is not a natural product, but is made by way of a manufacturing process known as hydrogenation. Food producers hydrogenate food to tailor the texture of the product, so that it is appealing to the masses (e.g., margarine that is spreadable). According to the *Dietary Guideline for Americans* (2005) students should learn to: Limit saturated fat consumption to less than 10% of their daily calories:

- Limit cholesterol consumption to less than 300mg per day;
- Keep trans fat consumption to as low as possible;
- Limit total fat consumption between 30 to 35 percent (for children two to three years-old) and between 25 to 35 percent (for youth four to 18 years-old) of their total calories intake; and
- Limit fat consumption as much as possible to sources of polyunsaturated and monounsaturated fats, such as fish, nuts, and vegetable oils.

Carbohydrates. Carbohydrates are also an important part of a healthy diet, and it is recommended that they make up 45 to 65 percent of total calories (Dietary Guidelines for Americans, 2005). Students can be taught that dietary fiber, simple sugars, and starch are carbohydrates, and they body breaks down the sugar and starch turning them into calories for energy for vital organs and muscles (Rizza, Go, McMahon, & Harrison, 2002).

Sugars are naturally found in foods like fruit and milk and can be added to foods. As it implies, added sugars are sugar and sugar-based products that are added during or after the processing or preparation of an edible item. Often on an ingredient list sugar may appear as: corn sweetener or syrup, dextrose, fructose, fruit juice concentrate, glucose, honey, lactose, maltose, malt syrup, molasses, and sucrose (Cafazzo, 2005). Added sugars are calorie-filled, yet contribute no or very little nutrients (Dietary Guidelines for Americans, 2005). Rizza and his colleagues (2002) explain:

> Foods that are high in added sugar are often low in essential nutrients such as vitamins and minerals. Unfortunately, these foods are often eaten in place of more nutrient-rich foods such as fruits, vegetables, and low-fat whole-grain products, and they may prevent us from obtaining essential nutrients and lead to weight gain. (p. 19)

While sugar and starch are digested into glucose and later used for energy, fiber – the non-digestable carbohydrate – is not. In fact, it does very little to provide energy (Kircshman & Nutrition Search, Inc., 2007). In the structure of the plant, fiber is the outer layer of a seed and the indigestible, tougher skeletal parts of plants (such as the skins of fruit and vegetables). It is regarded as the natural digestive system cleanser that helps maintain a healthy colon by laundering away substances that can lead to cancer and other digestive problems (Rizza et al., 2002). Students can learn these facts and that fiber gives the sense of satiety, which can help reduce overeating. Some believe that increasing the fiber in the diet of youth can help control childhood obesity. Kimm (1995) writes:

> Fiber-rich goods generally supply fewer calories and speed transit time through the digestive tract, and water-soluble fiber blunts the insulin response to carbohydrates. Also, fiber-rich diets tend to be carbohydrate-rich and low in fat. Increasing dietary fiber in children's diets could be a preventative measure with some study having show modest benefits for using dietary fiber in treating childhood obesity. (e1)

Cholesterol. The wax-like substance known as cholesterol is neither a fat nor does it provide any form of energy through calories, but is essential to our bodies. The liver in humans and animals produce enough cholesterol the body needs, but humans who eat animal products (e.g., meats, eggs, poultry, dairy, and so forth) intake excess cholesterol, which is often stored as plaque in arteries. Fruit and vegetables without added animal-based products do not contain cholesterol because they do not have livers). Too much cholesterol increases the risk of heart disease because plaque build-up blocks arteries that can lead to a heart attack or stroke. Cholesterol is often found in the foods that are high in saturated fat, which is concerning. Kircshman and Nutrition Search, Inc. (2007) expand, "The major dietary factor that increases blood cholesterol levels is saturated fat that the body is able to use to manufacture cholesterol. Dietary saturated fat has a greater impact on blood cholesterol levels than dietary cholesterol" (p.149).

Protein. Protein is not only found in foods but throughout all parts of the body including hair, nails, and teeth. Protein is pretty powerful, working efficiently by way of enzymes, antibodies, hemoglobin, and hormones (Bauer, 2005), and is a critical element for the vitality of a number of body components (Kirschman and Nutrition Search, Inc., 2007). The body breaks protein down into amino acids that are vital for bone, muscle, cartilage, skin, and other bodily functions (Ward, 2005). The body produces some amino acids, but it needs the remaining from foods we eat. Rizza (2002) and his colleagues underscore, "Protein is an essential part of our diets....Adequate protein is critical for growth, metabolism, and health, but eating more protein than we need will not build bigger muscles. Conversely, excess protein is converted to fat" (p.23).

Sodium. Because salt is sodium chloride, it is generally listed in the ingredient panel (on packages) as sodium. According the *Dietary Guidelines for Americans* (2005) most Americans consume more salt that their body needs, up to five to 18 times more, which is concerning because its intake in high quantities can negatively affect blood pressure leading to coronary heart disease, stroke, congestive heart failure, and kidney disease. The natural salt content in most foods is about 10% of total intake, added salt during personnel food preparation accounts for another 5 to 10%, but manufacturers add up to a whopping 75% (Dietary Guidelines for Americans). It is particularly important to teach students to read the sodium content on ingredient panels because some manufacturers add more salt than others on comparable products. The *Dietary Guideline for Americans* (2005) specifically suggest that it is particularly important to teach students to limit their sodium consumption to less than 2,300mg per day.

Calcium. Calcium is essential for a number of bodily functions but is particularly crucial for healthy teeth and bones. Calcium has long been associated with dairy products and many food manufacturers have capitalized on the idea that the body needs calcium for the development and maintenance of bone structure and rigidity (Kirschmann & Nutrition Search, Inc., 2007). Research has also established that calcium helps reduce the risk of high blood pressure and colon cancer (Gassenheimer, 2007).

Many laypersons inaccurately assume that calcium consumption is not as substantial to the body in adult life as it is in childhood and adolescence; however, calcium is needed throughout the lifetime. Our bodies store calcium in bones and whenever there is not enough calcium intake, the body takes it from them (Rizza, et al., 2002). In fact, calcium deficiency can lead to osteoporosis. Dairy products are a great source of calcium, but some have little or no calcium and are high in calories such as cream cheese, butter, cream and so forth. So, it is important that youth learn to consume calcium through dairy products and some food items such as salmon, sardines, oranges, almonds and tofu.

Iron. Nearly 70% of iron can be found in the hemoglobin area of red blood cells that transport oxygen in the blood (Bauer, 2005). When there is iron deficiency, there is little oxygen getting around to certain bodily functions, which can cause feelings of fatigue, shortened attention span, decreased work capacity, and impaired cognitive performance (Massey-Stokes, 2002).

Potassium. Potassium consumption is particularly critical because potassium-rich diets weaken the effects of salt on blood pressure and can reduce the risk of developing kidney stones (Dietary Guidelines for Americans, 2005). Kirschmann & Nutrition Search, Inc. (2007) elaborate, "Potassuim plays a vital role in many body functions, including muscle contraction, nerve transmission…potassium also helps keep skin healthy, protects against bone loss because of potassium's alkalizing effect in the body, and helps prevent kidney stones" (p.75). The recommended potassium consumption for adolescents is 4,700mg daily, 3000mg (for one to three-year-olds), 3,800mg (for four to eight-year-olds), and 4,500 (for nine to 13 year olds).

Vitamins. Vitamins are essential for many body functions, and depending on the vitamin can be particularly beneficial for: releasing energy throughout the body; supporting the nervous system; helping build body tissue; promoting good vision, healthy skin, and normal growth; maintain your bones, teeth, and mucous membranes (Ward, 2005; Bauer, 2005). Because the *Dietary Guidelines for Americans* (2005) mentions that children and adolescents in general have low intake of some minerals and vitamins, students should learn to eat foods that are vitamin rich or learn the best supplements to meet their unique needs.

2) Promote foods that ensure proper nutrition. As students learn about nutrients and other food substances, they should be encouraged to eat the right foods and avoid others. After all, youth are not born with an innate ability to choose a nutritional diet (Fuhr & Barclay, 1998). In general, youth will not make healthy choices unless they are exposed to nutritional foods and taught about them. Contemporary children and adolescents have low consumption of calcium, potassium, fiber, magnesium, and vitamin E, which suggest that they do not eat enough whole grains, fruit, vegetables, or drink or eat enough dairy products (The Dietary Guidelines for Americans, 2005). Ergo, efforts should be made to promote the importance of increased intake of foods that are rich in these nutrients. In fact, one of the Healthy People 2010 goals is to modify how Americans consume fat, calcium-rich foods, fruits, vegetables and grains.

One of the primary tasks is to help students understand that their diet choices contribute substantially to their health. Draw their attention to what they eat, how often, and why. Then explain that specific foods and beverages exist that are authentically healthy, while others may seem that way because they are marketed as low-fat, fat-free, and healthy when in fact they are high in calories, sodium, or are nutrient-inferior. In fact, research has found that some children have deduced incorrect nutritional beliefs from exposure to food ads (Robinson & Kullen, 1995).

An exceptional tool to promote nutritionally essential foods is the USDA pyramid guide. The federal government released the first Food Guide Pyramid in 1992 replacing the food wheel and the four basic food groups (Fuhr & Barclay, 1998). The Pyramid has become the most recognized and promoted nutritional guide in the nation. It is intended to help Americans (two-years-old and older) establish and maintain a healthy eating pattern of the right balance among the five food groups everyday. It is not meant as a temporary guide for rapid weight loss, but as a permanent way-of-life approach to healthy eating (Barlow & Dietz, 1998). The most current pyramid (January 2005), *MyPyramid* found in Figure, is comprised of grains, vegetables, fruits, milk, and meats and beans. While oil is not a food group, it is in the spectrum considered for good health and can be derived from fish, nuts, and corn, soybean, and canola oil.

MyPyramid reflects the latest nutritional science found in the 2005 Dietary Guidelines for Americans, and is intended to meet each person's unique dietary needs through different eating plans depending on their age, gender, height and weight, and physical activity level. The youth version, *MyPyramid for Kids* (Eat Right. Exercise. Have Fun.), and the adult version, *MyPyramid* (Steps to a Healthier You), instructs how much food from each of the food groups – in terms of servings in ounces and cups – to have for a specific calorie-diet. At the MyPryamid.gov website – by way of the *MyPyramid* Plan button – visitors can create a personalized plan for maintaining their weight or aim toward a healthier one.

Additionally, *MyPyramid* recommends:

Figure 4. MyPyramid[ii]

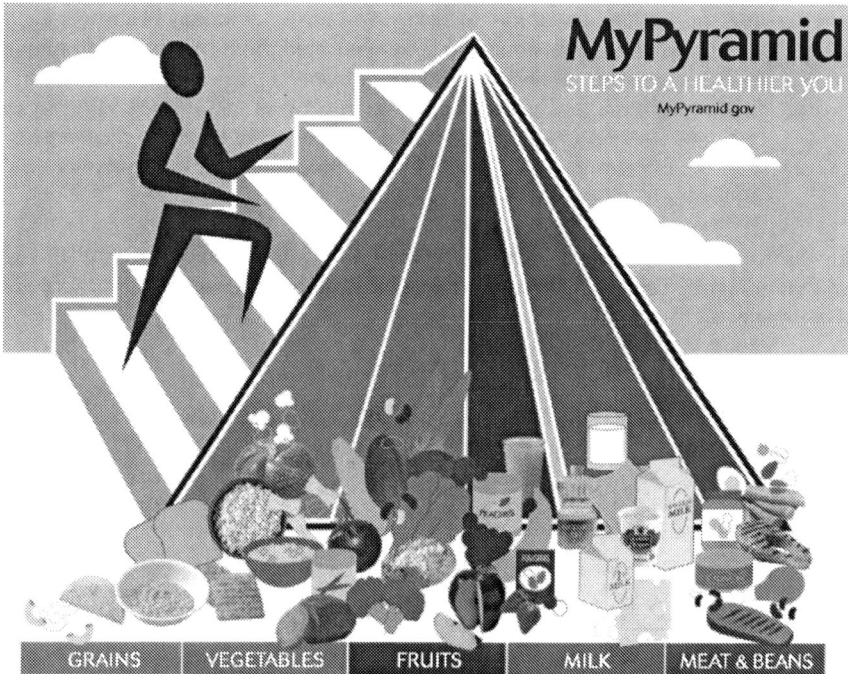

- Make most of your fat sources from fish, nuts, and vegetable oils.
- Limit solid fats like butter, margarine, shortening, and lard, as well as foods that contain these.
- Check the Nutrition Facts label to keep saturated fats, trans fats, and sodium low.
- Choose foods and beverages low in added sugars. Added sugars contribute calories with few, if any, nutrients. (U.S. Department of Agriculture, n.d., brochure)

Tips for youth are more specific:

1. Make half your grains whole. Choose whole-grain foods, such as whole-wheat bread, oatmeal, brown rice, and lowfat popcorn more often.
2. Vary your veggies. Go dark green and orange with your vegetables – eat spinach, broccoli, carrots, and sweet potatoes.
3. Focus on fruits. Eat them at meals, and at snack time, too. Choose fresh, frozen, canned or dried, and go easy on the fruit juice.
4. Get your calcium-rich foods. To build strong bones, serve lowfat and fat-free milk and other milk products several times a day.

89

5. Go lean with protein. Eat lean or lowfat meat, chicken, turkey, and fish. Also, change your tune with more dry beans and peas. Add chickpeas, nuts, or seeds to a salad; pinto beans to a burrito; or kidney beans to soup.

6. Change your oil. We all need oil. Get your nuts from fish, nuts, and liquid oils such as corn, soybean, canola, and olive oil.

7. Don't sugarcoat it. Choose foods and beverages that do not have sugar and caloric sweeteners as one of the first ingredients. Added sugars contribute calories with few, if any, nutrients. (U.S. Department of Agriculture, 2005, brochure)

An assortment of *MyPyramid* and *MyPyramid for Kids* resources are available at MyPyramid.gov. Table 13 illustrates elements from a downloadable brochure on how to meet the five food groups.

Table 13. Ideas from a MyPyramid brochure[iii]

Grains *Choose whole grains*	Vegetables *Go for the colors*	Fruits *Fresh, frozen, canned, and dried will do*	Milk *Feed your bones with high- calcium foods*	Meats & Beans *Go lean*
Have popcorn for a snack.	Dip baby carrots and green pepper strips in low-fat dressing.	Sprinkle raisins on breakfast cereal.	Make a smoothie by blending low-fat yogurt and frozen strawberries.	Add red kidney beans to a tossed green salad.
Make a peanut butter sandwich on whole wheat bread..	Try a salad made with spinach.	Have a frozen 100 percent juice bar for dessert.	Top a baked potato with low-fat cheese.	Sprinkle peanuts over stir fry vegetables.
Try oatmeal for breakfast.	Make black bean dip.	Carry an orange or apple in your backpack for snack.	Dip fruit in flavored yogurt.	Ask for boiled or grilled meat and chicken.
Snack on toasted oat cereal.	Bake a sweet potato in the microwave oven.	Snack on canned mandarin oranges.	Drink orange juice with added calcium.	Snack on soy nuts.
Have brown rice instead of white.	Order a veggie pizza.	Have a fruit salad for lunch.	Try soy milk or soy yogurt.	Take the skin off chicken.
Dip baked tortilla chips in salsa for a quick snack.			Drink plain or chocolate low-fat milk with meals.	Sprinkle nuts on frozen yogurt.
				Have tuna salad sandwich on whole wheat bread.

3) Incorporate activities that promote self-regulating behaviours. At this point, encourage students to exercise autonomy by self-regulating their consumption and setting limits on their choices (Strock, et al., 2005). Use *MyPyramid* resources to frame the message that non-nutritious foods abound in society and they are often associated with positive qualities (a cheese-burger, fries, a large Coke, a milk shake, a toy prize, a clown, colorful décor, and playground collectively do not exactly yield feelings of disgust or distress) and are palatable, but they are not healthy, and if consumed consistently over time can lead to lasting and irreparable physical harm. Underscore that although it may seem more expensive and less convenient to consume healthier products than packaged snacks, sweets, and soft drinks, a healthier diet lends itself to a better quality of life.

Teach students to restrict less healthful foods, control portion size, and choose better alternatives. To that end, consider implementing some activities that are fun, interactive, and relevant, and lead to healthful eating, such as:

Expose students to a variety of healthy foods. Bring in assorted nutritional foods into the classroom and hold tasting parties or taste tests. Have them see and taste foods from the various food groups, and foods that may be unfamiliar to them such as chickpeas, papaya, and so forth. Researchers have found that children have to try a food ten times before they accept it (Deckelbaum & Williams, 2001).

Grow a school garden. Have students plan for, plant, and maintain a garden of vegetables and fruit, which can be sold in the school cafeteria or used in the preparation of class meals. Such an activity affords them the opportunity to learn the nutritional value of herbage.

Help them select the right foods. Teach them to compare the foods they like. Have them compare: popular breakfast cereals with the healthier ones; cookies and candies with fruit; soft drinks with fruit flavored water, juices, and soy milk; and so forth. In other words, help them seek out nutritional alternatives to the popular foods, snacks, and beverages they know.

Help them understand their control over food selection. Teach students that even when nutrient-inferior foods are presented to them, they can select healthier options. Help them understand that they can enjoy sweets and pastries or colas, but in proper proportions. Underscore that they can eat burgers, fries, pizzas and other popular foods in moderation, with healthier ingredients, or in controlled portions. Insist that they too can become stewards of good healthy eating by teaching others (particularly parents, family members, and friends) about healthier foods and portion control. Incidentally, Linda Gassenheimer's (2007) book does an excellent job of teaching readers how to use their hand (e.g., palm-size, fist-size, two-finger portions) as a portion-size guide. Also, empower them to look and ask for more nutritious foods when they are grocery shopping with their parents.

Teach them to keep a food intake diary. Students can learn to record their food and beverage intake and determine how their diets compare to the *MyPyramid* guidelines. They can then assess how to modify their daily and weekly consumption so that it is healthier. Essentially, this teaches self-monitoring skills, which can help students change maladaptive behaviors (e.g., snacking while watching TV).

Discourse the benefits of water. Have the students research the benefits of drinking water, and then discuss water as a healthy alternative to colas, juices, and other soft drinks. According to Kirschmann and Nutrition Search, Inc. (2007), "Water is essential in dissolving and transporting nutrients such as oxygen and mineral salts via the blood, lymph, and other bodily fluids. Water also keeps the pressure, acidity, and composition of all chemical reactions in equilibrium" (p. 85). Then have the students brainstorm ways to replenish daily water loss.

Teach them about the nutrition facts label. The nutrition facts label allows persons to know the nutritional content of a product. Teach students to routinely read the labels paying specific attention to serving size and servings per container. For instance, two bags of cookies could very well indicate that a serving has 300 calories, but one serving size could be two cookies while the other could be ten. Eating ten cookies of the first bag would mean a consumption of 1,500 calories; eating ten cookies from the second bag would mean an intake of 300 calories. Students need to learn that labels offer calorie, fat, and other critical nutrient information that can help them make informed decisions in planning for a healthy diet. As a note of interest, research has found that label readers had diets that were lower in fat and higher in fruit and vegetable consumption compared to nonreaders, and others have noted that labels help youth avoid fad diets (Misra, 2002).

Encourage them to eat three well-balanced meals a day and snack less often. Skipping a meal can leave them hungrier later and looking for less healthier foods in the day (Cafazzo, 2005). Additionally, students with empty stomachs are likely to have a hard time concentrating and have very little energy, which can contribute to learning problems in the classroom.

Lastly, conduct these activities and other health promotions with considerable respect and forethought to the students' culture and socio-economic status. Understand that parents may not have the resources to buy healthier foods, or the time to prepare healthy meals for their children. In the lives of many families today, an economical meal is not necessarily the healthiest, yet it is not a parent's intent to deny their child well-balanced meals. Parents who only have two dollars to spend on their children's dinner will not look to the $2 bag of broccoli, but instead to bargain items that combined such as wieners, white bread, and generic chips.

Other families may not live in areas that have high quality foods with a wide selection. The nearest store may be a bodega with a limited selection of nutritious foods. Keep in mind that in some cultures being fit and thin is not a priority and many believe that a child with excess weight is the sign of healthy child. For many, frying most of their meals and eating sugar-laden pastries is commonplace. For youth from these types of cultures it is critical that parents receive notice about healthy diet lessons ahead of time and given literature about why healthy foods and healthy eating are important to overall wellness. Follow with some healthy, inexpensive meal plans and snacks for them to consider for their children. In many instances, parents will need nutrition education themselves.

Physical Activity and Exercise

Of course children and youth can maintain a healthy lifestyle by adhering to a well-balanced, nutritious diet as designated in MyPyramid. However, exercise is critical for their health and well-being. The benefits of exercise are abundantly clear: it keeps the pounds off; contributes to healthier bones, muscles, and joints; and has an excellent effect on insulin, blood pressure, and cholesterol levels, which helps reduce the overall risk of diabetes, blood pressure diseases, and cancer (Perry, 2004; Center for Disease Control, 2007). One study of 23 eight year-olds found that exercise had a positive effect on the blood flow of children's heart arteries. Prior to the study obese children had reduced blood flow compared to their normal-weight counterparts. After an eight-week exercise program, the blood flow through the obese children's heart arteries had improved significantly (Watts, Beye, Siafarikas, O'Driscoll, Jones, Davis, & Green, 2004). In short, exercise decreases the overall risk of developing chronic diseases later in life.

Primary physical activity goals for youth is to have them understand and accept that an active lifestyle is essential to their lives and to engage them in daily exercise. Teach youth that there are substantial gains to exercising. One study found that nearly half of students who watched a video on exercising and its affect on the cardiovascular system felt they were capable of improving their heart health (Levin, Martin, McKenzie, & DeLoise, 2002). Then, follow with current, developmentally appropriate practices in physical education (PE) instruction through a sequential kinder through senior year curriculum that is based on the National Association for Sport and Physical Education and the respective state standards. Underscore that physical activity is about health, not necessarily weight control.

Students should regularly receive age-appropriate PE taught by enthusiastic, board certified teachers who are quintessential role models of health and fitness. The wide-range of PE skills and concepts – fitness, sports, games, sportsmanship, gymnastics, and so forth – and actual PE engagement experiences should be designed to help students develop a lifetime affinity for and commitment to physical activity. Consequently, PE activities should not be strenuous or intense because students will develop a negative association with exercise. Instead the physical activities should be fun and enjoyable, yet moderate to vigorously challenging enough so that students learn to incorporate them into their daily lives. (See Table 14 for a glimpse of activities that are vigorously challenging). A 45-

minute game of kickball may be fun for some students, but it is not an aerobic activity when most of the students stand in field waiting for a ball that never comes their way. Research has found that only a small minority of children has daily PE, and their active class time is far below 50% (Datar & Sturm, 2004). In fact, 14% of all youngsters report no recent physical activity (Center for Disease Control, 2005). One 2000 study even found that only 8% of elementary schools, 6.4% of middle schools, and 5.8% of high schools have daily PE for the entire school year for all students in each grade (Institute of Medicine, 2004). These kinds of findings have led some to health experts to deem contemporary PE programs substandard and of limited value.

Table 14. Examples of moderate amounts of physical activity[iv]

Sporting activities	Common chores	
Playing volleyball for 45-60 minutes	Washing and waxing a car for 45-60 minutes	Less vigorous, more time
Playing touch football for 45 minutes	Washing windows for 45-60 minutes	
Walking 1 ¾ miles in 35 minutes	Gardening for 30-40 minutes	
Shooting baskets for 30 minutes	Pushing a stroller 1 ½ miles in 30 minutes	
Bicycling 5 miles in 30 minutes	Raking leaves for 30 minutes	
Fast social dancing for 30 minutes	Walking 2 miles in 30 minutes	↕
Water aerobic for 30 minutes	Shovelling snow for 15 minutes	
Swimming laps for 20 minutes	Stair climbing for 15 minutes	
Playing a basketball game for 15-20 minutes		
Bicycling 4 miles in 15 minutes		
Jumping rope for 15 minutes		
		More vigorous, less time
Running 1 ½ miles in 15 minutes		

To ensure that schools fulfill the nationally recommended 60 minutes of daily physical activities, students should also receive exercise through:

Daily recess. All elementary school children should be given at least 15 minutes to engage in free, supervised play. Encourage students to engage in moderate to vigorous exercise by providing them safe space and equipment. Recess should occur in the outdoors as often as possible.

Subject area lessons. Teachers should try to incorporate physical activity into their lessons. When appropriate, engage the students in some form of exercise. For instance, use exercise to teach math concepts (e.g., averaging) or take the students on a campus walk to get ideas about essay writing. Or, when the students seem dreary, take a break and play a game of kick ball.

School-sponsored celebrations. Have the school sponsor a full day event that promotes fitness where the students engage in a series of age-appropriate games, organized sports, and other recreational endeavors like obstacle courses. On that day, invite community members to teach students a sport that is rarely offered at their developmental level such as golf, archery, and so forth.

Before- and after-school programs. Offer students supervised extracurricular opportunities focused on physical activity such as organized sports, exercise, or martial arts classes. If enough students express an interest, sponsor a physical activity club (e.g., the runners club), intramural or interscholastic sports program, or develop a self-monitoring reward program that motivates students to engage in a physical activity, such as walking, and earn points toward an award. (See the President's Challenge Physical Activity and Fitness Awards Program discussed in Chapter One). In addition, if the school already has an after school program that supervises children until their parents are able to pick them up, encourage the caretakers to initiate some physical activities.

Lastly, because children become more sedentary as they grow older, PE instructors should teach students about the pitfalls of sedentary behaviors. They can point out how TV viewing and technology-use is attractive, but can lead to weight gain and other serious problems if they engage in these consistently for long periods of time. Moreover, PE instructors and all school personnel should encourage as much physical activity at school as possible, including doing household chores that are energy expending such as: raking leaves, shoveling snow, cutting the grass, and so forth.

Meals and Foods Served During the School Day

The school food service is an ideal learning laboratory for healthy eating where teachers can extend their instruction in practical ways. Toward that end, all schools should strive to improve the nutritional quality of what they sell and serve as part of their breakfast and lunch program and through other school-related activities, particularly fundraisers.

Many students meet their nutritional needs through the USDA National School Lunch Program (NSLP), which was signed into law in 1946 through the School Lunch Act (42 USC 1751). As written, the law is intended "to safeguard the health and well-being of the Nation's children and encourage the domestic consumption of nutritious agriculture commodities" (Taylor, 2003, p. 64). Essentially, the program was established to serve children living in poverty and suffering from malnutrition with a meal so that they could learn more efficiently in the classroom. Today, this federal program has grown into one of the largest feeding programs in the world with nearly 97,000 schools participating. In all, about eight million children (13% of the school-aged population) participate in the School Breakfast Program, and another 28 million (51%) participate in the NSLP.

Some researchers have found that federal school meals are compliant with the dietary guidelines providing 30% or less of the calories from fat (Lacar, Soto, & Riley, 2000), but others have noted that the meals are less than adequately healthful. Lynn-Garbe and Hoot (2005) explain:

> While school lunches in 1998-1999 had fewer calories from total fat and saturated fat than in previous years, they still, on average, were found to exceed the levels for total fat and saturated fat that are considered healthful. Children who participate in these meal programs have been found to consume higher amounts of fat and saturated fat in a 24-hour period than children who did not participate in the program. (p.72)

Strock and colleagues (2005) add:

> A survey study evaluating lunches in 500 schools in the US has shown that most schools serve meals that average more than 37-40% of their calories from fat. Only 1% of the 500 surveyed schools fell within the recommendations of American Academy of Pediatrics, US Department of Agriculture, and American Heart Association. (p. 21)

A larger problem is the food that is sold during lunchtime, which directly competes with the federal meals. Schools often sell competitive foods – foods and beverages that supplement the federal meals – as an alternative to relieve some of the operation costs since school meal services are financially self-supporting. According to the Center for Disease Control (cited in Coles 2004), nearly 43% of elementary schools and close to 90% of middle and 100% of high schools have a special school store or vending machine where students can purchase such competitive foods or beverages. One Cornell University researcher found that of elementary school cafeterias, 97% sold ice cream during lunchtime, 70% sold cookies or snack-cakes, and 46% sold chips (Human Ecology, 2003). Students, especially in high school, consume a significant portion of their daily calories from these competitive foods, which is unfortunate because often these foods are highly processed, high in fat or sugar, and low in other nutrients (Institute of Medicine, 2004).

To counter these two big problems, schools should offer foods that are affordable and appealing, yet meet the students' nutritional needs. This can be accomplished by convening a nutrition advisory council comprised of parents, students, nutritionists, teachers, and other administrators and assigning them the task of improving the quality of foods consumed at schools. The council could study the foods and adjust the menu items accordingly so that they comply with the USDA nutrition standards and support and reinforce the Dietary Guidelines for Americans. The council could ensure that the students: consume enough protein, iron, calcium and vitamins by way of whole grains, vegetables, fruit, low-fat dairy products, etc.; limit their intake of cholesterol, certain fats, sodium, sugar, and so forth; are served portion sizes that are age appropriate. As a guiding tool, the council could use the USDA "Prescription for Change: Ten Keys to Promote Healthy Eating in Schools," which is found in Table 15. Additionally, there are a number of things that schools can do encourage students to choose the healthier foods. Namely:

Offer healthy snacks and healthy drinks as a la carte items in the lunch line.
Here is the perfect opportunity to encourage students to consume healthier products like soymilk, bottled water, freshly cut vegetables, cups of fresh fruit, low-fat yogurt, and so forth. It might not be a bad idea to restrict the unhealthy snacks altogether, because one Baylor College of Medicine found that students in schools where snack foods were available consumed 50% less fruit, juice, and vegetables than their counterparts who did not have such access (Vail, 2004).

Price the healthy foods so that they are more affordable than the unhealthy counterparts. Students are likely to choose two chocolate cookies over a banana when they are both priced at a $1.00. One University of Minnesota study found that sales of carrot sticks and fresh fruit increased two to fourfold when the school cafeterias sold these at half price (Cowley et al., 2000).

Introduce a healthier or vegetarian option line. Have a special venue for students to eat baked, instead of fried foods, or a salad bar of fresh vegetables and fruit. Ideally, the cafeteria can offer a food stand where students can try foods that they may not readily have at home, such as: brown rice, spinach salad, baked sweet potato, vegetarian pizza or sandwich, tofu or tofu products like tofu ice cream or yogurt, soy nuts, and so forth.

Post the nutritional information and calorie count for meals, snacks, and beverages. When students know the nutritional value of foods, they are more likely to make informed decisions about what they eat, especially after having learned that some foods are better than others.

Table 15. Prescription for change: Ten keys to promote healthy eating in schools[v]

---

1. Students, parents, food service staff, educators and community leaders will be involved in assessing the school's eating environment, developing a shared vision and an action plan to achieve it.

2. Adequate funds will be provided by local, state and federal sources to ensure that the total school environment supports the development of healthy eating patterns.

3. Behavior-focused nutrition education will be integrated into the curriculum from pre-K through grade 12. Staff who provide nutrition education will have appropriate training.

4. School meals will meet the USDA nutrition standards as well as provide sufficient choices, including new foods and foods prepared in new ways, to meet the taste preferences of diverse student populations.

5. All students will have designated lunch periods of sufficient length to enjoy eating healthy foods with friends. These lunch periods will be scheduled as near the middle of the school day as possible.

6. Schools will provide enough serving areas to ensure student access to school meals with a minimum of wait time.

7. Space that is adequate to accommodate all students and pleasant surroundings that reflect the value of the social aspects of eating will be provided.

8. Students, teachers and community volunteers who practice healthy eating will be encouraged to serve as role models in the school dining areas.

9. If foods are sold in addition to National School Lunch Program meals, they will be from the five major food groups of the Food Guide Pyramid. This practice will foster healthy eating patterns.

10. Decisions regarding the sale of foods in addition to the National School Lunch Program meals will be based on nutrition goals, not on profit making.

Limit bake sales and fundraisers that sell candies or other baked goods. Fundraisers are notorious in schools, especially among clubs looking for money to travel or for new equipment. Often, students will strategically set up a table of baked goods in high traffic areas like the cafeteria, while others market chocolates or other candy (students can now raise money by selling frozen pies!) to the school population. These kinds of fundraiser are seemingly harmless, but they still avail nutrient-inferior foods to young people. In addition, these kinds of fundraisers send an indirect message that adults think it is OK to consume such nutrient-inferior products. Instead of selling donuts, brownies, and other sugary treats, school personnel should seek out alternatives such as selling organizers, calendars, Christmas cards, and so forth.

Restrict the sell of carbonated soft drinks and offer healthier alternatives.
Soft drink consumption among adolescents concerns many health experts because cola-type drinks constitute the leading source of sugar in their diet exceeding the daily-recommended limit (Human Ecology, 2003). Some data suggest that as many as 75% of teen males drink three cans of soda a day, while their female counterparts drink two (Covington et al., 2001). The calories alone, which are about 150 a can, easily add up to 300 to 450 calories a day, 2100 to 3150 a week not to mention that they have no vitamins and very few minerals (the diet ones can contain high doses of sodium and caffeine). While federal regulations already prohibit the sale of soft drinks during breakfast and lunch, schools are allowed to sell these after school and at their concession stands. But instead of offering cola-type beverages, why not offer healthier alternatives where students are compelled to drink them? Of course, the youngsters may very well go home and gulp down a cola or two, but by reducing the availability of these kinds of beverages they might learn that beverages such as these are enjoyed in moderation.

Restock the vending machines with healthy products.   Some schools offer students competitive foods by way of vending machines, which are often stocked with sugary snack foods and beverages. Schools that rely on these convenient revenue-producing vendors, however, can restock them with nutritiously healthy foods and beverages. Replace the chips and the candy with snacks like granola bars, fruit, etc. and offer flavored milk and water instead of the soft drinks. If this is not an immediate option, post the products' calorie nutritional value and calorie count so that the students can use this information in making their decision.

HOW SHOULD I APPROACH MY STUDENTS WHO ARE OVERWEIGHT OR OBESE?

While you may not have students in your classroom who are overweight or obese, with the rise in childhood obesity you most likely will. Thus, there may come a time when you ask yourself, "How should I treat this delicate issue? And, should I say something to the student, the parents, or both?" The sensitivity of the matter is enough to drive you to avoid the topic altogether, which is an option that many educators take. However, if school personnel sidestep the excess weight issue, many youth nationwide will continue to believe that there are no detrimental effects to being overweight or obese. Thus, as an educator you are obligated to address the issue by teaching the recommended healthy eating and physical activity habits that are outlined in the previous section and through supportive and encouraging actions and dialogue.

Students who are excessively overweight know better than anyone else that they are different from their peers. They know that they are overweight because they regularly compare themselves with others in school, in public, and in the media, and many peer groups single them out using words like fat, blimp, pig, Shamu, and so forth reinforcing the notion that their body size is a stigma. Consequently, many overweight youth come to school conscientious of their size.

Because youth generally base how they feel about themselves on how others treat them, it is especially important for you to convey that they are valuable, important, highly regarded, and special despite their girth and body size. They need your acceptance, understanding, and support, which you can indirectly model to other students, so that they feel good about themselves. Convey to all students that their physical features like weight and body-size do not shape the kind of person they are or how much you appreciate and respect them. You can say statements like:

- "In my eyes, it does not matter if you are tall, short, skinny, pudgy, black, brown, white, or orange, or that you wear braces or glasses, or that your hair is short, curly, or long, I appreciate you and do not judge you by your physical features."
- "Some of you think you look or talk silly, or feel awkward, or different than everyone else, but I and other appreciate who you are for your unique qualities."
- "Your family and school love you even though you might think you're too tall, too short, too skinny or too fat. Your physical features do not define who you are."

Toward this end, consider teaching lessons focused on the merit and advantage of diversity blended with messages of respect, acceptance, and tolerance of individual differences. In the vein that you teach about the equitable treatment and social justice of groups historically marginalized such as persons of color, persons with disabilities, women, and so forth, underscore that a person's size should also not matter in how they are perceived and treated. Also, consider teaching a lesson on the damaging effects of stereotypes because many youth may think that their overweight counterparts are lazy or lack willpower. Stress that size, like color of skin, gender, physical limitations, sexual orientation, and so forth do not completely define a person, his ability, or capability. Lastly, inform the students that you do not tolerate any form of insults or epithets or bullying and teasing in the school, including those that are body-size based. Of course this makes for a safer school environment, but it also sends the powerful message that no one should be made fun of. If you hear or see abuse of any kind, be sure to immediately reprimand the offender and reassure both parties that weight or body size does not diminish a person's character and strengths.

The question remains, should you say something directly to the student? Foremost, never single out the child with a statement like, "I noticed that you are bigger than the others. Is there something you would like to talk about?" Or, "I'm a little concerned because you're looking chubbier than usual." And, "Have you been eating extra helpings of grandma's cooking?" Reportedly, one teacher patted a boy's stomach and said, "Too many tamales, Jorge!" Even though you may have all the sincerity in your heart and voice, approaches like these are likely to hurt or embarrass the student and perhaps cause irreversible emotional damage. Youth who carry excess weight would want to crawl under the nearest desk after hearing these kinds of comments. No good can come from criticizing or blaming the student for their excess weight. Instead, address the whole class with positive comments about healthy eating and physical activities, teach some of the discussed recommendations in the previous section, and encourage all students to try new physical activities and healthier foods. Whole group instruction is far more desirable than a pull-aside.

At no time suggest that students go on a diet, especially one that deprives them of nutritious food like a water diet. As aforementioned, the goal for youth is to adopt lifelong habits that embody a healthier and active lifestyle. When the opportunity presents itself share your testimony about healthy eating and the physical activities you engage in or enjoy. You can encourage students through your own adventures casually suggesting they can do the same. For instance, you can say:

- "This weekend I washed my car by hand and then I took my dog for a very long walk. It was great exercise."
- "It was really tough to get myself to go for a jog, but I felt so good afterwards."
- "Ask your parents if they can take you to the park down the street. There is so much room to play different sports. I played a game of basketball with a couple of the guys there."
- "Who wants to be in my exercise club? You have to promise to do the same amount of exercise just like I do after school, and then we encourage each other in the morning."

A student who approaches you with concerns about their weight is quite a different affair. You should be honored if this happens. The student evidently trusts you and believes that you can help. Understand that the student has mustered up considerable courage to bring this to your attention, so take the situation very seriously. You should:

1. Listen.

Listen to what the student has to say. Be sensitive to the idea that they may feel stigmatized by their peers or distressed about their appearance. If they are visibly upset, allow them the time to regain their composure. Other students may be fine with their weight and body-size and are simply seeking for your advice on how to lose weight. Either way, in a private setting you can ask developmentally appropriate probing questions that allow them to express their feelings, such as:

- "How long have you been feeling like this?"
- "Did someone say something to hurt you?"
- "How have you been handling this?"
- "Have you talked this over with someone else?"
- "What have you done to work this through?"

Listen the whole time and interject as little as possible.

2. Offer Support.

Offer additional support by reaffirming that their character and unique qualities are not defined by their weight status. Relate that they are an OK person at any weight by underscoring their positive qualities. Follow with statements that suggest how difficult it must be to worry about weight at their age. You can validate their feelings with comments such as:

- "It must be tough, especially when you look at the magazines and the pictures show so many unrealistically skinny celebrities."
- "I can understand why this is hard for you. It's hard for me whenever I see adults my age who have ideal bodies."
- "Sometimes we are so hard on ourselves when we don't look like the actors on TV or the people around us. It's enough to drive anyone crazy."

3. Informally Assess Their Diet and Physical Activity.

At this point, ask them about their daily eating habits and physical activities. Probe for specific signs of unhealthy patterns, such as a diet of too much fried foods, minimal exercise, and so forth. It is important that your questions intimate you care and that you do not judge them. Start by asking their permission to inquire into their life. You can ask, "Is it okay if I ask you a couple of questions about your health habits?" Or, "Do you want to talk about this?" Then carry on with questions such as, "Is it okay if we start with your BMI and the daily fat and calorie count you should have?" Or, "What do you eat on a daily basis? Let's map out your meals and try to solve how many grams of fat or calories total for the day." And, "How much exercise do you get in a day?" In other words, examine their wellness behaviors such as those discussed in the prior section. Then, follow with questions focused on: the family's history of weight or attitudes and behaviors toward food/meals; medical conditions associated with weight gain; and psychological issues (e.g., eating disorder). If you suspect a medical or psychological problem, immediately refer the student to the nurse or school psychologist, especially if the student is depressed.

4. Ask If They Want Your Help.

Some students may only want to vent and seek your support, but others may come hoping you can help them get on track toward a healthy lifestyle. For those who want help offer them healthy suggestions based on the information outlined in the prior section. This is a great opportunity to sit down with them and make a plan for healthy eating and daily exercise, as well as one for what they can say to their parents. Start off with simple suggestions (e.g., reduce the sugars, drink more water, walk for 20 minutes, etc.) and work toward more challenging objectives. Be sure to outline physical activities that are not too difficult or could cause them some embarrassment. Additionally, suggest that the student keep a diary, which can track progress and later be used to modify the plan. Give them healthy lifestyle brochures and resources (see Chapter 7) for them to later read, and if they are amenable, enlist the school coach and district nutritionist for specialized help. Remind them that the goal is not about weight loss, but about being physically, mentally, and socially healthy. As a caution, do not plan for ambitious or aggressive efforts because a reluctant or unready student will be left with a damaged self-esteem, and future attempts to improve his or her lifestyle will be bleak.

5. Encourage.

Energize and enhearten the student. Emphasize that the student can maintain a healthy and active lifestyle. If you are open to the idea, suggest that the two of you begin living healthier lives together by keeping tabs on each other's progress, or start an after—or before—school exercise club for all students. Encourage the student to return to talk to you, and celebrate the accomplishments, even if they seem small to you (e.g., walking 20 minutes for three days in a row). Ultimately, let him know that you are available for continual support.

If you have a student who is morbidly obese and you strongly believe that his health is in imminent peril because he has difficulty breathing, sleeping, or experiences sorts of pain, or if he is socially withdrawn and depressed, then talk to the school nurse, school psychologist, counselor, and social worker about intervening with him and his parents in private. Mention how the professional team is concerned about the affect his body weight and size have on his physical well-being. Give special thought to what you say so that he or his parents (who may also be overweight or obese) are not humiliated or offended. Start by asking if they perceive that their child has a weight problem, and ascertain if they believe that it affects his health. Then, educate the parents about the importance of healthy eating and physical activity, which can occur over a series of informational meetings. Carefully explain some of the adverse effects of having excess weight. Segue by resolving whether they are willing to fully support him in a healthy diet and exercise plan, and what help and information they will need in order to make it happen. All the while, express care and concern as the rationale for the intervention.

Every situation is uniquely different, so the team should determine on a case-by-case basis whether the student should be in the meeting. If he shows some reluctance, then having him there may cause him undue hardship. However, if he seems receptive to the idea, invite him accordingly and solicit information about what his challenges might be and his willingness to enter a health-centered program. The team can certainly develop a healthy eating and exercise plan with a counseling component for continuous support, but strongly advise the parents to first take him to their pediatrician for a complete medical evaluation. The doctor can recommend a weight management program for youth and/or refer him to a certified nutritionist for further diet consultation. Ultimately, the team can work with doctor and nutritionist to get the student on a healthy track. All the while, stress to parents that they should accept and love their child at any weight, not treat him any differently than they do their other children, and encourage (not nag or criticize) him to strive for a healthy lifestyle.

Parents are in the optimal position because they can make suitable changes in their child's diet, encourage accordingly, and model a health lifestyle. In the event that you are concerned about other overweight and obese students, send home information and brochures to all the parents about eating right and exercise. Many parents will not fully understand that a child's excess weight can be detrimental to their physical, mental, and social well-being, so be prepared to answer a myriad of questions and follow with suggestions.

CONCLUSION

Given that schools reach over 56 million youth and adolescents; they make for an efficient childhood obesity solution. Schools can systematically educate students on the multiple dimensions of wellness while promoting nutritional and exercise practices that can shape their attitudes and behaviors for a lifetime. In due course, students can learn and develop effective decision-making skills that steer them toward eating well-balanced meals and nutritious snacks and engaging in a healthy work out. This can be accomplished in a number of ways through a coordinated school health program that empowers students with the knowledge and skills to make responsible choices. Such programs are comprehensive with a planned, sequential curriculum that incorporates national standards, federal and state guidelines, best instructional practices, and encompass health, physical, and nutrition education. If you have students in your classroom who are overweight or obese, rather than a pull-aside discussion, teach the whole class how to maintain and improve their health and how to reduce unhealthy practices and behaviors. If a student is morbidly obese or you have others whose health concern you, gather a committee of school health professionals to discuss the matter with the student's parents. What to say and suggestions to offer the parents and the family are further discussed in the next chapter.

NOTES

[i] Source: U.S. Department of Agriculture. (2007). Local wellness policy: Frequently asked questions. Retrieved April 22, 2007, from http://www.fns.usda.gov/tn/Healthy/wellnesspolicy_faq.html.

[ii] Source: U.S. Department of Agriculture. (2007). MyPyramid. Retrieved April 22, 2007, from http://www.fns.usda.gov/tn/Healthy/wellnesspolicy_faq.html.

[iii] Source: University of Missouri Extension. (n.d.). Adapted from USDA publication CNPP-15. Columbia, MO: Author.

[iv] Source: Adapted from U.S. Department of Health & Human Services. (2007). *Being physically active can help you attain or maintain a healthy weight.* Retrieved April 7, 2007, from http://www.surgeongeneral.gov/topics/obesity/calltoaction/fact_whatcanyoudo.htm.

[v] Source: American Obesity Association. (2007). *Childhood obesity.* Retrieved April 14, 2007, from http://www.obesity.org/subs/childhood/prevention.shtml.

REFERENCES

American Dietetic Association, Society for Nutrition Education, & American School Food Service Association. (2003). Position of the American Dietetic Association, Society for Nutrition Education, and American School Food Service Association: Nutrition services: An essential component of comprehensive school health programs. *Journal of Nutrition Education & Behavior, 35(2),* e20.

Baranowski, T., Cullen, K., Nicklas, T., Thompson, D., & Baranowski, J. (2002). School-based obesity prevention: A blueprint for taming the epidemic. *American Journal of Health Behaviors, 26(6),* 486-493.

Barlow, S., & Dietz, W. (1998). Obesity evaluation and treatment: Expert committee recommendations. *Pediatrics, 102(3),* e11.

Barlow, S., Trowbridge, F., Klish, W., & Dietz, W. (2002). Treatment of child and adolescent obesity: Reports from pediatricians, pediatric nurse practitioners, and registered dieticians. *Pediatrics, 110(1),* e14.

Bauer, J. (2005). *Total nutrition* (Fourth edition). New York: Alpha.

Brownlee, S., Martens, E., McDowell, J., & Sieger, M. (2002). Too heavy, too young. *Time, 159(3),* e3.

Cafazzo, D. (2005). *Fighting childhood obesity: A long way to go.* Retrieved March 2, 2005, from http://www.thenewstribune.com/news/local/v-printer/story/4634495p-4301726c.html.

Carmona, R.H. (2003). *Remarks to the 2003 California Childhood Obesity Conference.* Retrieved February 18, 2007, from http://surgeongeneral.gov/news/speeches/califobesity.htm

Center for Disease Control. (2005). *Adolescence and young adults.* Retrieved April 12, 2005, from http://www.cdc.gov/nccdphp/sgr/adoles.htm

Center for Disease Control. (2007). *Prevalence of overweight among children and adolescents: United States, 1999-2002.* Retrieved April 2, 2007, from http://www.cdc.gov/nchs/products/pubs/pubd/hestats/overwght99.htm

Coles, A. (2004, May/June). Generation XXL: Obesity among U.S. schoolchildren is on the rise, and schools can help fight this battle of the bulge. *American Teacher,* pp. 6-7.

Covington, C., Cybulski, M., Davis, T., Duca, G., Farrell, E., Kasgorgis, M., Kator, C., & Sell, T. (2001). Kids on the move: Preventing obesity among urban children. *American Journal of Nursing, 101(3),* 73-81.

Datar, A., & Sturm, R. (2004). Physical education in elementary school and body mass index: Evidence from the Early Childhood Longitudinal Study. *American Journal of Public Health, 94(9),* 1501-1506.

Davis, S., Davis, M., Northington, L., Moll, G., & Kolar, K. (2002). Childhood obesity reduction by school based programs. *ABNF Journal,* 145-149.

Deckelbaum, R., & Williams, C. (2001). Childhood obesity: The health issue. *Obesity Research, 9(4),* e7.

Feeg, V. (2004). Combating childhood obesity: A collective effort. *Pediatric Nursing, 30(5),* 361-362.

Fowler-Brown, A., & Kahwati, L. (2004). Prevention and treatment of overweight in children and adolescents. *American Family Physician, 69(11),* 2591-2598.

Fren, M., Malin, S., Bansal, N., Delgado, M., Greer, Y., Havice, M., Ho, M., & Schweizer, H. (2003). Addressing health disparities in middle school students' nutrition and exercise. *Journal of Community Health Nursing, 20(1),* 1-14.

Fuhr, J., & Barclay, K. (1999). The importance of appropriate nutrition and nutrition education. *Young Children, 53(1),* 74-80.

Gassenheimer, L. (2007). *The portion plan: How to eat the foods you love & still lose weight.* London: DK Publishing.

Graf, C., Koch, B., Kretschmann-Kandel, E., Falkowski, G., Christ, H., Coburger, S., Lehmacher, W., Bjarnason-Wehrens, B., Platen, P., Tokarski, W., Predel, H., & Dordel, S. (2004). Correlation between BMI, leisure habits and motor abilities in childhood. *International Journal of Obesity, 28(1),* 22-26.

Hardy, L. (2004, September). Congress requires school wellness plans. *American School Board Journal,* pp. 6-14.

Harris, K. (2002). The USDA school lunch program. *Clearing House, 75(6),* e4.

Horodynski, M., Hoerr, S., & Coleman, G. (2004). Nutrition education aimed at toddlers: A pilot program for rural, low-income families. *Family Community Health, 27(2),* 103-113.

Human Ecology. (2003, December). Preventing childhood obesity at school, at home, and in the community. *Human Ecology*, p. 23.

Institute of Medicine. (2004). *Schools can play a role in preventing childhood obesity.* Retrieved July 20, 2007, from http://www.iom.edu/Object.File/Master/22/615/Fact%20Sheet%20-%20Schools%20FINALBitticks.pdf.

James, D., Rienzo, B., & Frazee, C. (1997). Using focus groups to develop a nutrition education video for high school students. *Journal of School Health, 67(9)*, 367-379.

Kirschman, J., & Nurtrition Search, Inc. (2007). *Nutrition almanac: Fight disease, boost immunity, and slow the effects of aging* (Sixth edition). New York: McGraw Hill.

Lacar, E., Soto, X., Riley, W. (2000). Adolescent obesity in a low-income Mexican American district in South Texas. *Archives of Pediatric & Adolescent Medicine, 154(8)*, 837-840.

Levin, S., Martin, M., McKenzie, T., & DeLoise, A. (2002). Assessment of a pilot video's effect on physical activity and heart health for young children. *Family & Community Health, 25(3)*, 10-17.

Massey-Stokes, M. (2002). Adolescent nutrition. *Clearing house, 75(6)*, e11.

McArthur, L., Pena, M., & Holbert, D. (2001). Effects of socioeconomic status on the obesity knowledge of adolescents from six Latin American cities. *International Journal of Obesity, 25(8)*, 1262-12-68.

McMurray, R., Harrell, J., Bangdiwala, S., Bradley, C., Deng, S., & Levine, A. (2002). A school-based intervention can reduce body fat and blood pressure in young adolescents. *Journal of Adolescent Medicine, 31(2)*, 125-132.

Misra, R. (2002). Influence of food labels on adolescent diet. *Clearing House, 75(6)*, e8.

Neumark-Sztainer, D., & Story, M. (1997). Recommendations from overweight youth regarding school-based weight control programs. *Journal of School Health, 67()*, 428-433.

Perry, P. (2004, Nov/Dec). Putting the brakes on childhood obesity. *The Saturday Evening Post*, pp. 64-68.

Perez-Rodrigo, C., & Aranceta, J. (2003). Nutrition education in schools: Experiences and challenges. *European Journal of Clinical Nutrition, 57(S1)*, S82-S85.

Robinson, T., & Killen, J. (1995). Ethnic and gender differences in the relationships between television viewing and obesity, physical activity, and dietary fat intake. *Journal of Health Education, 26(2)*, S91-S96.

Strock, G., Cottrell, E., Abang, A., Buschbacher, R., & Hannon, T. (2005). Childhood obesity: A simple equation with complex variables. *Journal of Long-Term Effects of Medical Implants, 15(1)*, 15-32.

Stone, E., McKenzie, T., Welk, G., & Booth, M. (1998). Effects of physical activity interventions in youth: Review and synthesis. *American Journal of Preventative Medicine, 15(4)*, 298-315.

U.S. Department of Agriculture. (2005). *MyPyramid: Eat right. Exercise. Have fun.* Washington, DC: U.S. Department of Agriculture.

U.S. Department of Health and Human Services. (2005). *Dietary guidelines for Americans.* Retrieved March 9, 2007, from http://www.health.gov/dietaryguidelines/dga2005/document/

U.S. Department of Health and Human Services. (2007). *Overweight and obesity: A vision for the future.* Retrieved February 18, 2007, from http://surgeongeneral.gov/topics/obesity/calltoaction/fact_vision.htm

Vail, K. (2004). Obesity epidemic. *American School Board Journal, 191(1)*, 22-25.

Veugeler, P., & Fitzgerald, A. (2005). Effectiveness of school programs in preventing childhood obesity: A multilevel comparison. *American Journal of Public Health, 95(3)*, e10.

Ward, E. M. (2005). *The new food pyramid: Commonsense advice that demystifies the new nutritional guidelines.* New York: Alpha.

Watts, K., Beye, P., Siafarikas, A., O'Driscoll, G., Jones, T., Davis, E., & Green, D. (2004). Effects of exercise training on vascular function in obese children. *Journal of Pediatrics, 144(5)*, 620-625.

HEALTH PROMOTION AT HOME

Children did not create the obesity crisis that is afflicting their lives. Adults led the way by creating the fast food chains, eating and serving larger food portions, engaging in sedentary pastimes, popularizing unhealthy snacks, and so forth. With the rates of childhood obesity soaring, adults—especially parents – are implicated in the childhood obesity epidemic because they lead by example. They are therefore obliged to transform their attitudes toward food and exercise and work efficiently to reduce the risk factors that cause children to become overweight.

Because no parent dreams of the day that their child will grow up to be overweight, much less obese, it is reasonable to assume that parents are willing to learn how to alter their behaviors and home environment to engender a healthy child. There are numerous complicated influences in the home that shape children's eating and physical activity behaviors that lead to excess weight. Not to mention that children live in environments where they have very little or no control over what they eat; their parents do. Based on these circumstances alone, it is apparent that parents can become a positive force in the prevention and intervention of childhood obesity. Parents simply need the awareness that they can make a difference and the knowledge associated with promoting their children's health.

In this chapter, a discussion ensues in regard to these questions:
- Why should health promotion efforts involve parents and the family?
- How can parents and family members be involved?

WHY SHOULD HEALTH PROMOTION EFFORTS INVOLVE PARENTS AND THE FAMILY?

To reverse the increasing trend of childhood obesity, society will have to experience a socio-cultural transformation of sorts, which can occur in homes through parents and the family. American family life has changed dramatically in the last couple of decades. There was a time when children were raised in homes where mothers had time to prepare wholesome meals; where children played outside and rode their bicycles, and gathered around their fathers who helped with homework. This Norman Rockwell image that many of our elders lived and enjoyed is now reality for a few American families. The safety concern for children coupled with parents' work schedules, TV viewing habits, video game and computer usage, and other aspects of the modern day lifestyle has decreased children's opportunities for healthy meals and regular exercise. Despite these challenges, parents have to join forces with schools, public offices, and private industry to curb the escalating trend.

Parents share the responsibility to do something to protect their children's health because only a small dent will be made on the obesity crises if attention is focused solely on the school, for instance, or among public officials, or within the food industry and media. To illustrate this point, imagine a student who has been learning about nutrition and eating the right number of fruit and vegetables for his developmental age and body frame. His teacher reinforces the importance of eating right; he learns a nifty mantra, "Three out of five, healthy, and alive"; and, he eats a well-balanced meal at school. Subsequently, he is taught that being physically active is more desirable than sitting around. While all of this instruction is worthwhile, it benefits him little if he returns to a home where the family eats high fat, high-calorie foods and snacks, and lays around watching TV. In this mixed messages war, the family wins out because multiple family members can consistently reinforce and model that their way is the right way. Thus, prevention efforts without parent and family involvement does little good for children or social transformation.

Parents and family members should become involved in health promotion efforts because children learn lifestyle habits – often unhealthy ones – from them early in their childhood. Families are a powerful influence because they are the child's first major socio-cultural learning laboratory that teaches acceptable behaviors (Moran, 1999). Unsurprisingly, children grow to identify with and imitate familial behaviors, especially those of their parents (Chen 1996). Studies have found that family characteristics, particularly the general condition of the family, family lifestyle habits, and parental guidance, contributed significantly to children's overweight problems (Wu, Yu, Wei, & Yin, 2003). Thus, it is reasonable to assume that families must be educated and empowered about the impact they have in children's development of eating and physical activity habits. The nursing profession has long embraced this notion and actively engages families in their health promotion programs. For instance, in weight management programs, practitioners seek to:

- increase a family's understanding about the matter;
- increase a family's ability to identify with behaviors incompatible with healthy living;
- promote an understanding of behavior modification; and
- promote an understanding of methods for behavior modification. (Drohan, 2002)

The entire family should be involved when carrying out health promotion because long-term research has shown that children keep the weight off when the prevention and intervention is aimed at the parents and the child, rather than the child alone (Moran, 1999). The authors of the *Time* magazine feature article on childhood obesity underscore that health programs have to entail families to be successful. In their interview with psychologist Leonard Epstein, director one of the most successful pediatric obesity programs around, Brownlee and colleagues (2002) underscore:

'You really need to include parents as part of the treatment,' he says, if only because parents of obese children are often overweight or obese themselves. Usually, the entire family could stand to modify its diet and reduce high-fat foods and sweets. (p.e3)

Parents are key figures in health promotion because their weight status is a reliable predictor of childhood obesity (Myers & Vargas, 2000). Some researchers have found that when one parent is obese, there is a 40% chance that the child will become obese, contrasted with 10% when neither parents is obese. The percentage leaps to 80% when both parents are obese (Zwiauer, 2000). The American Academy of Pediatrics (2003) reports that before a child is three years-old, parental obesity is a stronger predictor of adult obesity than the child' weight status. This leads the Academy to emphasize, "Such observations have important implications for recognition of risk and routine anticipatory guidance that is directed toward healthy eating and activity patterns in families" (p.425). This kind of information is important because even though there may be varying factors that are contributing to parents' weight status, it is highly likely that they are overweight because of their lifestyle, which ultimately has its affect on children.

As the Institute of Medicine (2005) points out, parents should be involved in health promotion programs because they are the child's teacher. They influence their children by modeling behaviors. They teach them about values, mold attitudes, and reward or reinforce children's behaviors. Parents are also the policy makers and policy enforcers constantly deciding what happens in or outside the home. Just as they safeguard their children from illegal substances, alcohol, and smoking, and curb their children from cursing, they too set the rules for the way the family eats and exercises. As the policy administrators, parents select and prepare the foods that shape their children's food preferences for a lifetime. Keep in mind that parents are also a banking system that dispenses allowances, which children use to purchase candies and other sugary snacks and soft drinks. Thus, when parents are involved in health promotion they can set the limits for acceptable behaviors.

Involved parents can help resolve the excess weight issue. Because they often do not recognize that their children have a weight problem, they could be making matters worse for their children. As Dennison (cited in Tucker, 2000) found, some parents feed their children based on the perception they have of their child's weight. Specifically, parents who do not identify their children as overweight (even when their children's BMIs are over the 85th percentile) are less likely to limit their child's overall food intake, and more likely to feed their children whole milk and use dessert as a reward. Indeed, research has found that parents generally do not see or accept the fact that excess weight is a health issue for their children. Myers and Vargas (2000), for instance, found that nearly 35% of parents did not perceive that their obese child was overweight when in fact they were. Jain, Sherman,

Chamberlain, Powers, and Whitaker (2001) discovered that mothers described their overweight children as "thick" or "solid" if they had healthy diets and/or good appetites and were physically active. Interestingly, the times the mothers defined their children as obese were when they thought their children were teased or could not participate in physical activities. Some of the mothers also believed that they could not affect their child's weight because their children were predisposed to overweight, and some found it emotionally difficult to deny food to their child. Assumingly, some parents may deny the weight problem because they believe that the child will outgrow the excess weight or out of fear that they will offend their children and make matters worse. Others may not see a problem with the excess weight because their cultural belief about body status that perceives nothing wrong with a heavyset child. Or they may avoid the topic altogether because they too have a longtime weight problem. Regardless of the reasons, if parents do not fundamentally perceive that excess weight is a problem, then it makes sense that they be involved and given the tools to address the issue with their children. Otherwise, their children will continue on the path of excess weight gain.

HOW CAN PARENTS AND FAMILY MEMBERS BE INVOLVED?

Parents and family members can take a comprehensive course of action when they become involved in health promotion at home. Namely, they can guide the family by making long-term, lifestyle behavior changes with respect to diet and nutrition, and regular physical activity. Additionally, they can focus their attention on health and well-being, not quick, inadequate weight loss methods that are potentially harmful to children's development. To effectively involve parents, they must be educated with the knowledge that they can make long-lasting changes that lead toward healthful behaviors. The tools to facilitate these changes are grounded in what the U.S. Surgeon General Richard Carmona (U.S. Department of Health & Human Services, 2003) calls, health literacy. He defines health literacy as, "the ability of an individual to access, understand, and use health-related information and services to make appropriate health decisions" (p.e6).

In order for parents to make changes at home, they must first be informed as to what excess weight in childhood means. In other words, they need the childhood overweight and obesity crises brought to their attention in a sensitive, non-judgmental manner with specific recommendations on how to assess whether their own child is overweight. This is particularly important for two reasons. First, as aforesaid, many parents do not recognize or accept overweight in their children as a problem and can unknowingly foster unhealthy diets and behaviors. Second, children do not become overweight or obese on their own. They live in environments where they have very little control – where adults generally make all the decisions for them. Parents need to understand that just as they helped their children put on the pounds; they can also help shed them off.

Next, they must learn about the potential physical, mental, and social risks associated with overweight and obesity. Parents have to be taught that overweight children can develop high blood pressure, diabetes, high blood cholesterol, and other chronic diseases that alter quality of life. They must come to realize that overweight or obesity is a burden on children's emotions, self-esteem, and social status, which are closely tied to feeling subordinate to their normal-weight counterparts.

Lastly, they can be empowered with health-related information and specific ways to safeguard and support their children's health. This can be accomplished through an approach the Society for Nutrition Education (2003) terms, "Health at Any Size." The approach is health-centered, unlike the weight-centered methods that are aimed at reducing weight, and is focused on the well-being of the whole person. Translated, this means eating in healthy ways, living actively, and respecting persons at the size they happen to be. "Health at Any Size" has an emphasis on modifying lifestyle habits with the goal of having a healthy weight they define as, "the natural weight the body adopts, given a healthy diet and meaningful levels of physical activities" (p. 60). The Society opposes the concept of ideal weight because it can be unrealistic for some, which can confound matters. Adapting this approach for parents would suggest that they apply their acquired health-related information, specifically excess weight, eating attitudes and behaviors, physical activity, and body image by: 1) fostering a nurturing environment; 2) establishing healthful dietary behaviors; and 3) promoting and supporting opportunities for fun physical activities.

Fostering A Nurturing Environment

The Society for Nutrition Education (2003) stresses that parents create environments that encourage and sustain children on their journey toward healthy living. In a nurturing environment, parents acknowledge that their child has a weight problem and listen to what the child has to say. They talk to their children in a loving and supportive fashion paying careful attention not to place blame, sound critical, or make other comments that can erode their self-concept and esteem. Nothing can harm a child faster than a judgmental remark like, "You're starting to pork up because you eat too much," or "Take a good look at yourself." Because children often compare themselves to their peers, they know when their waist- and body-size is larger than most. And, if they are subjected to rounds of teasing or bullying at school, the last thing they need is their parents' reminder that they are fat. Instead, they need their parents' unequivocal acceptance – open and consistent expressions of love, praise, and positive feedback that set the stage for how they feel about themselves. Children need their parents' motivation to accelerate their journey toward health. Parents can also emphasize the importance of constructive values like character, aspiration, and so forth and discredit some of the media's obsession with appearance and the seemingly pervasive spotlight on the ideal body. Despite how some children and adolescents might respond on the outside to a hug or comment or two about how they are appreciated, internally they need the affirmation that their parents care about their well-being. The world is filled with characters that are ready to crush their spirits; they certainly do not need them in their own home.

Children with caring and supportive parents are more likely to feel good about themselves and better equipped to make lifestyle changes. These changes can begin by parents offering to work collaboratively with their children to set and accomplish realistic, achievable goals. The family is destined to make short-term gains: from temporarily joining a commercial gym that is cumbersome to get to on a regular basis; from nagging parents who make their children run a mile or two in the heat of the late afternoon; or from parents who require them to weigh in daily. Instead, parents should take a helpful, relaxed attitude, by offering, inviting and confirming ideas for family consideration, and then involving themselves in the suggested activities. Parents are wise to approach the ideas at a slow pace or one that is comfortable for their children, and praise them for trying new practices and making healthy behavior changes, even if they seem small. Parents can call attention to the positive changes – like when their child plays outside for 30 minutes instead of watching TV – and monitor themselves away from dwelling on or badgering about the bad ones – like when they catch their child sneaking a mouthful of chocolates. All the while, parents should attempt to gradually change the whole family's eating habits and physical activity routine and not single out one member from the others. As caution, a focus on weight reduction can backfire with untoward consequences, especially when there is a cycle of weight loss and gain. According to physicians Fowler-Brown and Kahwati (2004) weight loss is only recommended for overweight children who have medical conditions, but only under the advice and guidance of a family physician. Parents should instead concentrate on maintaining the child's current weight while they grow normally in height (Brown University, 2005).

In a nurturing environment, parents can set the example for making healthy changes. Children develop long-term habits based on what they see their parents and family members doing. So, if they regularly witness a parent choosing healthy foods and active pastimes, their children will do the same. When they see the positive associations, listen to their parents discuss the inherent benefits, and accept their parents' invitation to accompany them like a buddy, then they are more likely to change their ways.

Establishing Healthful Dietary Behaviors

Parents can influence children's eating practices by setting the rules and the norms as they relate to food. They can help young children develop positive perceptions, attitudes, and behavior toward food and eating, and can guide their children toward making healthy choices during meals and snack times. They can further improve their children's eating behavior by following these healthful suggestions.

Assess children's eating habits. With as much help of their children as they are capable, parents can determine what their children eat, when, and how often. Over a week or so, they can survey daily routines to ascertain behavioral patterns and estimate the amount of calories their children consume. Parents can identify the specific foods that are eaten regularly and whether they are high in fat, calories, or sugar, or are nutritionally inferior, and then adjust how often they avail these to children. Later, parents can introduce self-monitoring logs where children keep a daily diary of the foods they consume. Such a diary exposes the good and bad eating habits, which yield to later progress evaluation and behavior modification (Drohan, 2002).

Teach about healthy eating practices. Parents can directly inform (or learn with) their children on how to best meet their nutritional needs. They can read about the essentials for daily nourishment, foods that are particularly beneficial for children's growth and development, and foods that offer little nutrients but are appealing because they are savory (e.g. cakes, pies, etc.). Parents can talk to health professionals like the school district nutritionist, their family practice physician, or a clinical dietitian, and ask for healthy eating recommendations. Parents can impart this knowledge to their children by helping them make food choices that follow the suggestions and the MyPyramid guidelines as well. They can also review the key recommendation noted in the *Dietary Guidelines for Americans* (U.S. Department of Health & Human Services, 2005):

- Make smart food choices from every food group;
- Find balance between food and physical activity;
- Get the most nutrition out of your calories; and
- Know the facts, use the food label. (Loyo, 2006, p. 19)

At some point parents can interject a message about the importance of safe food handling practices, which are outlined in Table 16.

Table 16. Safe food handling practices[i]

The Dietary Guidelines for Americans outlines these key food safety recommendations:
To avoid microbial foodborne illness: • Clean hands, food contact surfaces, and fruit and vegetables. Meat and poultry should not be washed or rinsed; • Separate raw, cooked, and ready-to-eat foods while shopping, preparing, and ready-to-eat foods while shopping, preparing, or storing foods; • Cook foods to a safe temperature to kill microorganisms; • Chill (refrigerate) perishable food promptly and defrost foods properly; and • Avoid raw (unpasteurized) milk or any products made from unpasteurized milk, raw or partially cooked eggs or foods containing raw eggs, raw or undercooked meat and poultry, unpasteurized juices, and raw sprouts.

Avoid fad and restrictive diets. Parents can examine the damaging effects fad or restrictive diets have on children. It is important that parents and children understand that healthy eating is a permanent lifestyle change, not a temporary one with the goal of weight loss. Children need healthy doses of food for daily living and severely cutting back on what they eat can interfere with their growth and development. It is best that parents offer their children a balanced diet with a variety of foods in smaller portions and have their children choose what they want to eat. This particularly important because children often have to try a food 10 times or more before they accept it (Cafazzo, 2005), and some health experts believe that it is easier to learn to like all foods during the first five or six years of life than it is later in life (Fuhr & Barclay, 1998).

At some point, parents can take the opportunity to discuss the notion of moderation. Parents should let their children know that they do not intend to abruptly deny them the foods they are accustomed to and love (like sweets), but that the treats and other favorites will be made available within reasonable limits. Otherwise, the children will begin plotting on how to consume them without their parents finding out. To illustrate this point, one Texas schoolteacher reported that one of her second grade students loved ice cream, but was told by her mother that she could no longer have any more because she was looking chubbier than her peers. Unbeknown to the teacher and the mother, for nearly two weeks during lunch the youngster bought an ice cream cone on credit. When the $8 tab came due, her enraged mother asked how she planned to get away with the scheme, to which the daughter replied, "I was always thinking of ways I could pay the lunch lady back."

Teach about media influences. Parents can also talk to their children about the influence media has on promoting nutritiously inferior products such as sugary snacks and soft drinks or fast foods that are often fattening. Research suggests that TV viewing correlates with children's caloric consumption and food request. Some have found that the media even influences children to request their parents to buy particular foods (Proctor, et al., 2003). Borzekowski and Robinson (2001) believe that preschool youngster's exposure to one or two 10 to 30 second food commercials can effect their short-term preferences for specific food products. To help children understand marketing tactics, parents can collaborate with their children and examine some of the products that are highly promoted, especially those showcased during popular kid shows. Together, they can look at how product campaigns, design, and convenience affect consumer buying power, and then compare the nutritional values of products against MyPyramid, *Healthy People 2010*, or the *American Heart Association Dietary Guidelines*. If the children still long for specific products, parents can buy them along with healthy alternatives as long as they review the idea of moderation. There is an excellent website, www.fatcalories.com, that allows web visitors to ascertain the calories, fat, and other nutritional components of the menu items found at fast food chains. Parents can use this as a tool to teach children to avoid the wrong foods and discredit media messages. Collectively, this can help limit the purchasing and subsequent intake of foods that provide few nutrients.

Avoid using foods as a comfort or reward. To further develop their children's healthy attitude toward foods, parents are wise to refrain from using food as a comfort or reward. Of course foods are meant to be enjoyed, but not at the cost of developing dreadful habits. For instance, when distressed children are comforted with food, they may come to learn that certain foods—generally savory, high calorie treats– are a source of consolation, and later in their adulthood may revert to heavy doses of ice cream, chocolates, and so forth whenever they find themselves in a dilemma. Parents should teach children how to deal effectively with their feelings (e.g., discuss their frustrations with others, take a hike to relieve stress, and so forth) instead of turning to overeating when they become emotional. Using food as a reward or bribe produces similar effects. When parents promise one food for another they inadvertently impart that one is superior to the other. So if dessert is offered only when the child eats all his vegetables, he learns that vegetables are not as important or as delicious as dessert and will learn to prefer the more valuable of the two (Brownlee, Martens, McDowell, & Sieger, 2002).

Respect children's appetites. Parents should respect their children's appetite and never force them to eat everything off their plate. Research suggest that children are born with an innate ability to recognize when they are full, but they grow to ignore these internal cues because they are conditioned to completely finish their meals (Brownlee, et al., 2002). Thus, parents are inadvertently harming their children when they insist that they eat everything that is presented to them. Instead, parents should enhance their children's ability to detect satiety by encouraging them to stop eating when they are full, instructing them to not eat when they are not hungry, and coaching them to eat slowly to detect feeling full (Broadwater, 2002). This is parents' golden opportunity to discourage their children from eating in front of the television because it can be difficult to attend to feelings of satiety when they are distracted by the programming and – not to mention – can lead to overeating (National Institute of Health, 1997). Some researchers have noted that a decrease in the number of meals eaten in front of the television produces significant reductions in the BMI and skin-fold tests of boys and girls (Dennison, Erb, & Jenkins, 2002). As often as possible, the family should eat together engaging in conversation and enjoying the meals in designated areas of the home – like the kitchen and dining room – away from the television (National Institute of Health). When the mealtime and conversations are pleasant and relaxed, the children are more likely to eat slower and develop positive associations with eating.

Involve children in meal planning and grocery shopping. Parents can give children a role in the family's decision making by allowing them to help with the meal planning and grocery shopping (Broadwater, 2002). Parents can reinforce nutritional concepts by working with their children to combine and prepare foods to produce healthy meals and to explore alternative snacks that are most beneficial for energy (McArthur, Anguiano, & Gross, 2004). By assigning them preparation, serving, and clean-up duties, children are more likely develop a sense of accomplishment and a willingness to try and eat foods they had a hand in arranging (National Institute of Health, 1997). Research suggests that children want to be involved in these kinds of family-based activities. According to McArthur and colleagues, children know that good dietary practices are important and want their parents to help them make good food choices.

Read food labels with children. Food labels are meant to guide consumers in their diet planning. Parents can work with their children to read food labels to learn about the nutritional content of foods they intend to consume. Together they can use the label information to choose the foods that are beneficial and consistent with *Healthy People 2010* or the *Dietary Guidelines for Americans*, and avoid those that are not. Food labels are great tools to help parents and their children make informed decisions. They can use them when they want to snack (e.g., compare the nutritious content of low-fat cookies with pastries), quench their thirst (e.g. compare a soft drink with a juice), and plan a meal (e.g., compare fettuccine Alfredo with a skinless chicken salad). And in the times they want to indulge in nutrient-inferior products (in moderation, of course), they can adjust their diet accordingly. After all, parents and their children do not have to stop eating any one food altogether, but decrease the portion size and the frequency of those foods when they can. See Table 17 for a description of the food label components.

Respect culture. Because ethnic culture is mainstay among many families with unique dishes having an expected place on the dining room table, parents have to work with their children to subsume the foods into their adopted healthy meal framework. Many families have regular preferences for the ethnic dishes, which are often high in calories and fat, and will undoubtedly have a difficult time separating from them. As an example, there are many Mexican American families who eat refried beans and tortillas daily. To ask families to give these up would be like stripping them of their identity. To resolve the issue, parents can lead a discussion about the significance of their dishes and follow closely with recommendations on how to alter them so that they can be enjoyed regularly. They can then reassure the family that the dishes in the customary recipe will be enjoyed in moderation, like on special occasions or cultural holidays.

Buy healthy foods and prepare healthy meals. As often as they can, parents should buy healthy products that lend themselves to healthy meals for their families. When they shop at the grocery store, parents and their children should look for foods that balance the five major food groups (including the oils needed for good health) found on MyPyramid. As Loyo (2006) advises, they should seek out "vegetables, fruits, whole grains, and fat free/low-fat milk and milk products.... lean meats, poultry, fish, beans, eggs and nuts.... (and choose) foods that are low in saturated fat, trans fat, dietary cholesterol, salt, and added sugars" (p. 19). Moreover, they should buy foods that meet the national recommended daily allowance: two and half cups of vegetables with an emphasis on dark green, orange, legumes, starchy, and others throughout the week; two cups of fruit; three cups of calcium rich foods; and three ounces of whole grains. See Table 18 for some tips for following the *Dietary Guidelines for Americans*.

Table 17. Pointers parents and children can use from food labels[ii]

Serving Size

Is your serving the same size as the one on the label? If you eat double the serving size listed, you need to double the nutrient and calorie values. If you eat one-half the serving size shown here, cut the nutrient and calorie values in half.

Calories

Are you overweight? Cut back a little on calories! Look here to see how a serving of the food adds to you daily total. A 5'4", 138-lb. active woman needs about 2,200 calories each day. A 5'10", 174 lb. active man needs about 2,900. How about you?

Total Fat

Aim low. Most people need to cut back on fat! Too much fat may contribute to heart disease and cancer. Try to limit your calories from fat. For a healthy heart, choose foods with a big difference between the total number of calories and the number of calories from fat.

Daily Value

Feel like you're drowning in numbers? Let the Daily Value be your guide. Daily Values are listed for people who eat 2,000 or 2,500 calories each day. If you eat more, your personal daily value may be higher than what's listed on the label. If you eat less, your personal value may be lower. For fat, saturated fat, cholesterol and sodium, choose foods with a low % Daily Value. For total carbohydrate, dietary fiber, vitamins and mineral, your daily value goal is to reach 100% of each.

Saturated Fat

A new kind of fat? No – saturated fat is part of the total fat in food. It is listed separately because it's the key player in raising blood cholesterol and your risk of heart disease. Eat less!

Cholesterol

Too much cholesterol – a second cousin to fat – can lead to heart disease. Challenge yourself to eat less than 300 mg each day.

Sodium

You call it "salt," the label calls it "sodium." Either way, it may add up to high blood pressure in some people. So, keep your sodium intake low – 2,400 to 3,000 mg or less each day.

Total Carbohydrate

When you cut down on fat, you can eat more carbohydrates. Carbohydrates are in foods like bread, potatoes, fruits, and vegetables. Choose these often! They give you nutrients and energy.

Dietary Fiber

Grandmother called it "roughage," but her advice to eat more is still up-to-date! That goes for soluble and insoluble kinds of dietary fiber. Fruits, vegetables, whole-grain foods, beans and peas are all good sources and can help reduce the risk of heart disease and cancer.

Protein

Most Americans get more protein than they need. Where there is animal protein, there is also fat and cholesterol. Eat small servings of lean meat, fish and poultry. Use skim or low-fat milk, yogurt and cheese. Try vegetable proteins like beans, grains and cereals.

Vitamins and Minerals

Your goal her is 100% of each for the day. Don't count on one food to do it all. Let a combination of foods add up to a winning score.

Table 18. Tips for following the Dietary Guidelines for Americans[iii]

The new 2005 Dietary Guidelines are the blueprint for a healthy lifestyle. Reducing calories, making wiser food choices and exercising more are the keys. Specifically, you should: eat more nutrient-packed foods like low-fat or nonfat dairy foods, fruits and vegetables, and whole grains.

Low-fat or Nonfat Dairy
3 cups daily
1 cup = 1 cup of low-fat/nonfat milk or yogurt, 1 ½ ounces of low-fat or nonfat cheese
Tips
- Add a slice of cheese to a sandwich
- Stock up on string cheese and yogurts for lunches and snacks
- Start your day with dairy: whole grain cereal and milk or fruit and yogurt
- Make a smoothie with a cup of yogurt, your favorite, fruit and ice

Whole Grains
At leas 3 ounces whole grains
1 ounce = 1 slice of whole-grain bread, 1 cup whole-grain cereal, ½ cup of cooked brown rice or whole-wheat pasta
Tips
- Choose whole-grain breakfast cereal
- Use whole-grain bread or a roll for you sandwich
- Stock your pantry with brown rice and low-fat, whole-grain crackers
- Put some crunch in your yogurt by adding a whole-grain cereal or granola

Fruits and Vegetables
4 ½ cups fruits/vegetables
1 cup = 1 cup fruits/vegetables
1 large apple, 2 cups leafy salad greens
Tips
- Spruce up a sandwich by adding grated carrots
- Add a serving of broccoli or steamed vegetables at dinner
- When eating out, swap French fries for a serving of plain vegetables or a salad – even fast food restaurants now offer this!
- Enjoy vegetable sticks with low-fat yogurt dip, cottage cheese or hummus

---

Choose healthy snacks. Because snacks *are* an American way of life, parents and their children should seek out a variety of healthy alternatives instead of eliminating them altogether. After all, snacks help persons maintain an energy level between meals. A strategy might be to limit snacks in the house as opposed to stocking them in the cupboards and then restricting their access—forbidding them might make them seem all the more desirable (Brownlee, et al. 2000). As Gable and Lutz (2000) found, children will eat high sugar, high fat snacks if they are available in the home. As one Texas grocer advises, when it comes to snacks, parents can consider these healthful tips:

- Eat every 2-3 hours (snack when meals are more than four hours apart);

- Snacks are a bridge between meals; they are not meant to make you feel full; and
- Snacks should have a maximum of 100 calories (for a small frame person) up to 150 calories (for a larger frame person). (H.E. Butt Grocery Company, n.d., p. 2)

Parents should avoid buying the nutritiously empty snacks that are often pre-packaged, pre-prepared, sugary, and fried, and purchase and offer snacks like fresh fruit and vegetables, low-fat yogurt, fat-free cheese, small amounts of dried fruits, Graham or animal crackers, and so forth. See Table 19 for a host of healthy snacks. To help ease the blow of not getting the snacks that their children are accustomed to, parents can let them choose the healthy ones they find most appetizing. Because Americans consume about 30% of their calories from snacking, parents should consider limiting how often the family snacks (Institute of Medicine, 2004). Parents and their children can determine the best times in the day to snack without spoiling their appetites at mealtime. More importantly, they should remember to do so in designated eating areas.

Table 19. Some health snacks [iv]

One Texas grocer distributes a flyer of these recommended snacks	
Fruits	*Dairy*
Apples	Lowfat yogurt
Cherries	Lowfat cottage cheese
Dried apricots	1% or skim milk
Grapefruit	Mozzarella string cheese – part skim
Oranges	Lowfat soy milk
Peaches	
Pears	
Plums	
Prunes	
Proteins	*Combinations*
Hard-boiled eggs	Banana & peanut butter
Nuts – peanuts, almonds, walnuts,	Whole grain crackers & peanut butter
cashews, pecans, pistachios, soy	Whole grain bread & peanut butter
Sunflower and pumpkin seeds	Cottage cheese & fruit
Peanut butter	Raisins & peanuts
	Lean lunchmeats or tuna & crackers
	Celery & peanut butter
	Yogurt & granola
	High fiber cereal & milk
	Bread & cheese
	Yogurt & berries
	Pita & hummus
	Grapes & cheese
	Strawberries & Nutella

Monitor Portion Sizes. The portion sizes in the diet of many Americans are considerably overestimated. Young and Nestle (2002) found that the portion sizes of foods on Americans' plates are between 28% to 700% larger than what the USDA and Food and Drug Administration recommends. Indeed, it is not uncommon for some to eat a plate full of spaghetti when the suggested portion size is about the size of a computer mouse, or eat gobs of cheese when the recommended portion size is about the size of a domino. Linda Gassenheimer (2007) author of *The Portion Plan: How to Eat the Foods You Love & Still Lose Weight*, expands:

> A growing body of research shows that most people are blissfully unaware of how much food is being put in front of them. At Pennsylvania State University, research found that people tended to eat whatever was on their plate or in a serving package....the researchers found that adults ate at least 30 percent more calories when larger portions of these foods were put in front of them – even though they generally were just as satisfied by the smaller portion....Other studies using potato chips and candies have shown drastic increases in snacking when the subject was given a larger amount of food to dip into. (p. 12)

When parents and children eat large portions they make way for hundreds of extra calories that lead to excess weight. In fact, consuming an extra 100 calories a day for a year (without expending them through physical activity or exercise) can lead to a weight gain of 10 pounds. To counter this excess weight gain, parents should carefully cut down on the portion sizes of the foods they eat. Parents can start by serving the portions according to the needs of each family member then work their way toward suggested portion sizes. Gassenheimer's (2007) book, which uses the different parts of the hand (e.g., palm, fist, finer, thumb, etc.) to indicate ideal portion sizes, is an excellent resource to learn how to serve appropriate portions. Others recommend that parents think of everyday objects to determine portion sizes. For instance, the portion size of:

- a three-ounce serving of meat is equivalent to the size of a deck of cards;
- butter is the size of a die;
- cheese is the size of a domino;
- oil is the size of a quarter;
- medium fresh fruit is the size of a tennis ball;
- one cup of raw vegetables is the size of light bulb;
- ½ cup of ice cream is the size of tennis ball; and
- one cup of mashed potatoes is the size of a fist.

Encourage children to eat slowly. Parents and their children should avoid rushing through meals. Not only does eating fast increase the chances of choking and possible stomach afflictions, health experts believe that persons who eat fast have a difficult time detecting when they are full. For these reasons and more, nutrition consultants often encourage persons to eat slowly by taking smaller bites, chewing food longer, and putting down their utensils between bites (American Obesity Association, 2007b).

Limit eating out. Many families enjoy eating out. In fact, eating out is no longer for special occasions like the generations of yesteryear, but a way of life for many persons. As Unger and colleagues (2004) point out, nearly a third of the total calories consumed by Americans come from foods prepared away from home. Let's face it; eating out, especially at fast food restaurants, is convenient, affordable, consistent and offers an array of meal options to satisfy nearly all family members. It is no wonder that fast food restaurants are ubiquitous in our society. They are in food courts in malls, chain restaurants in and around shopping centers, and bistro-like versions in airports, truck stops, and Wal-marts.

While they might seem like a godsend to the busiest of families, there are some inherent disadvantages of eating out. In particular, the portion sizes are often larger than the USDA recommendations. Apparently when McDonalds first opened, a meal of their hamburger, fries, and Coke totaled 600 calories. Today, a meal of their Quarter Pounder with Cheese, Super Size Fries, and a Super Size Coke totals to 1,550 calories (smartmouth.org, 2007). Many of the chains even boast that bigger is better with slogans that embrace descriptors like: supersize, kingsize, value meal, supreme, biggie, and colossal. What they fail advertise is that bigger also means more fat, calories, sodium, cholesterol, etc. than the meals prepared at home. Gassenheimer (2007) admonishes, "The increase of size in fast food portions is one of the reasons we are fatter than ever before. Not only is the food often chockfull of calories and saturated fat, but we also eat it too frequently" (p. 13). Parents would break their family's spirit if they ruled that fast food or eating out was no longer an option. So, rather than initiate what could be their children's revolution against health altogether, parents should cut down on the number of times they eat out. When they do eat out, parents can guide their children into making healthier food choices, like choosing the healthier options from the menu items. The American Dietetic Association (1997) offers these tips for parents to balance the meals consumed outside the home:

- Order small servings of French fries, shakes and other high-fat foods;
- A grilled chicken breast or regular hamburger is a lower-fat choice than a deep-fried fish or chicken patty sandwich;
- Balance high-fat foods, such as French fries, chicken nuggets, or hot dogs, with low-fat foods at other meals and snacks throughout the day;
- Visit the salad bar with your children and let them pick out their favorite fruits and vegetables. Top the salad with low-fat salad dressing;
- If you eat out often, you could let your children choose French fries or another high-fat food on alternative visits. On other days allow them to choose a lower-fat substitute, such as spaghetti with meat sauce or pizza with mushrooms and olives; and

- Children often enjoy soup (broth-based) and bread sticks, appetizer-size or half-portions of main dishes, or meals composed of two or three side dishes. (brochure)

Ensure children eat breakfast every day. It might sound glib, but breakfast is a very important meal. Eating a well-balanced breakfast is an excellent start to the school day. Skipping it or skimping on it may leave children with less energy for concentration, which can affect their achievement. Moreover, children with empty stomachs are likely to look for and consume less healthy foods later in the day (Cafazzo, 2005).

Encourage children to resists sugary drinks. Sodas are pervasive in our society. Researchers have found that yearly soft drink production has increased from about 100 twelve ounce can per person in the 1940's and 1950's to approximately 600 cans per person in the 1990's (Jacobson, 2007; Gerrior, Putnam, & Bente, 1998). Soda drinking is particularly worrisome because sodas are loaded with sugar, which means they are high in calories. In fact, if a child drinks two 12-ounce sodas each day for one month, he would consume about a five-pound bag of sugar (Health EDCO, 2005). To avoid the excess calories gained from soda drinking, parents should offer their children water and other healthy drinks when they are thirsty, and discourage sodas and other sugary drinks including the fruit juice and sports drinks.

Parents should remember that children should drink milk regularly (nearly two to three cups a day) since it is source of calcium for their growing bodies. This is particularly important because as the *Dietary Guidelines for Americans* (U.S. Department of Health & Human Services, 2005) points out, "Milk product consumption has been associated with overall diet quality and adequacy of intake of many nutrients, including calcium, potassium, magnesium, zinc, iron, riboflavin, vitamin A, folate, and vitamin D" (p. 9). But rather than buy whole milk, parents should gradually switch from whole to skim (once their children are over two years-old) because skim milk does not have as much fat.

Promoting and Supporting Opportunities for Fun Physical Activities

Just as Americans could stand to eat healthier, they could use the exercise too. The rate of obesity is at an all time high not only because adults and children alike do not eat well, but also because they do not get the daily exercise or physical activity they need. The average American gains about 10 pounds each year, which could be reversed by expending just 100 calories a day (Hill, 2004). According to Carmona (U.S. Department of Health & Human Services, 2007a), 60% of Americans do not meet the minimum goal for physical activity, which is 30 minutes of moderate to vigorous activity on most days. This is why one of the leading *Healthy People 2010* objectives it to engage all people in regular physical activity.

This intention did not come by whim. Health experts recognize a number of physical, psychological, and social benefits that are associated with physical activity, which includes increased life expectancy and decreased risk of cardiovascular diseases (American Heart Association, 2007). Mandel (2007) points out that engaging in regular physical activity benefits "a healthy cardiac system, insulin regulation, bone and muscle building, core balance, as well as creating mental focus, self-esteem and empowerment" (p.e2). The American Heart Association specifically adds that physical activity reduces blood pressure, raises good cholesterol, and reduces the risk of diabetes and certain kinds of cancer. See Table 20 for a list of benefits that physical activity produces. Some health experts also believe that physical activity may be the most efficient way to prevent weight gain, to lose weight, or to keep it off (Broadwater, 2002, U.S. Department of Health & Human Services, 2007b). Consistent physical activity is particularly important for children because it leads to increased levels of alertness and attention, which is closely tied to their academic achievement (Lifelines, 2002). Regular physical activity in children's lives is advantageous all the way around. As professor of exercise and sports science at University of North Carolina Robert G. McMurray puts it, children who exercise regularly will likely live longer, healthier, and more satisfying lives (NewsRX, 2002).

Table 20. The American Heart Association Advertises The Many Benefits of Physical Activity [v]

Regular physical activity is an important component of a heart-healthy lifestyle. It "exercises" your heart muscle, promoting heart health. Combined with heart-healthy food choices, regular activity can:

- Reduce the risk of heart disease by improving blood circulation.
- Keep weight under control.
- Improve blood cholesterol levels.
- Prevent and manage high blood pressure.
- Prevent bone loss.
- Boost energy level.
- Help manage stress.
- Release tension.
- Improve the ability to fall asleep quickly and sleep well.
- Improve self-image.
- Counter anxiety and depression and increase enthusiasm and optimism.
- Increase muscle strength, providing greater capacity for other physical activity.
- Provide a way to share an activity with family and friends.
- Establish good heart-healthy habits in children and counter the conditions that lead to heart attack and stroke later in life.
- In older people, exercise can help delay or prevent chronic illnesses and diseases associated with aging and maintain physical agility and quality of life.

Because of the inherent health benefits associated with exercise, most health organizations like that American Heart Association, National Association for Sport and Physical Education, and the U.S. Surgeon General Carmona recommend that youth between five and twelve years-old spend at least an hour or more engaged in developmentally appropriate physical activity on all or most days of the week. In addition, parents should encourage their children to be active through play or other activities during the day. Moran (1999) advises, "Initial exercise recommendations should be small and exercise levels should be increased slowly, to avoid possible discouragement. A reasonable goal is 20 to 30 minutes of moderate activity per day, in addition to whatever exercise the child gets during the school day" (p. e8).

Here are some simple ways that parents can help their children on their road to an active lifestyle:

Assess children's current level of physical activity. Parents should determine the extent of exercise their children get regularly. Together they can add up how much exercise the children get on a daily basis to and from school, while at school, after school, and at home in the evenings and the weekends. This can include the times the children are in PE, in organized sports like T-ball or flag football, in free outdoor play, or doing chores around the house. This kind of assessment is important because it exposes the factors that stand in the way of children becoming physically active, which then helps parents adapt how they spend their leisure time. For instance, if the parents determine that their children could walk to school instead of being driven, they can adjust their morning routines to make the walk feasible. Or, if they notice that the family sits around on the weekends and watches TV, the parents can make plans for outdoor types of activities like a hike or swim at the community center.

Encourage children to engage in regular physical activity. Our environment is one comprised of appliances, gadgets, and modes of transportation designed to make life easy, comfortable, and pleasurable nearly everywhere we spend time. While modern day advances are amazing, they are also to our detriment because they cut into the amount of physical activity we exert. What is particularly worrisome is that modern day children are being raised in environments where so much is done for them, that physical activity is often perceived as more of a nuisance than an attractive means for health. Thus, parents have to mold their children into believing that physical activity plays a pivotal role in their lives. As often as possible, they should encourage their children to do something active. This can be accomplished by simply giving their children the opportunity to get involved in some sort of physical activity, whether it is by way of organized sports or assigning them household chores that are energy expending like washing the car or raking leaves.

Despite their individual differences, all children need physical activity in their lives. Parents should expose children to a range of activities that are appealing, which can cover light calorie burning activities (e.g., free play) and those that increase the heart rate like swimming, biking, jumping rope, skating and so forth.

Parents should seek out clever ways to get their children out of the house. For instance, they can:

- Make an obstacle course in the backyard and have families with other children come to participate;
- Adapt a popular board game to encompass physical activities;
- Make weights from plastic soda bottles filled with sand and schedule exercise time;
- Have a block party where the neighborhood children complete fitness tasks; and
- Introduce non-team sports like dance or the martial arts.

To further motivate their children, parents should make supportive comments whenever they see their children engaged in physical activity, even though the achievements may seem small. If they can afford to, they can also reward them with outdoor play equipment, fitness clothes, or special trips to the park, recreation center, or the nearest playground. Lastly, parents should encourage their children to try an organized sport that the school or community has to offer.

Find activities children prefer and enjoy. Children can be easily discouraged from physical activities that are not fun, as they will quickly grow to resent any exercise they perceive as a punishment. Parents should therefore look for physical activities that are age and developmentally appropriate. Children's bodies are not equipped to participate in exercise that is adult-based like using elliptical machines or treadmills; nor would most children want to be introduced to physical activity that requires them to run two miles, use the Stairmaster for 30 minutes, or lift rounds of weights. Based on their assessment of their children's fitness level, parents can start by having them try different activities, and narrow down those the children find most enjoyable. As they become more active, parents can intensify the ones the children enjoy or add more vigorous activities (Moran, 1999). All the while, parents should be sensitive to their children's' feelings and needs. Because some children are uncomfortable with their overweight bodies they will shy away from certain physical activities (Tremblay & Willms, 2003), so it is important that parents find physical activities that children will not find embarrassing or difficult (National Institute of Health, 1998).

Be a role model. Parents can do wonders by setting the example for their children. As role models, parents can lead their children toward becoming physically active by doing simple things like intentionally parking far away, climbing the stairs instead of using the elevator, working on the yard, and so forth, and working their way toward more elaborate activities like jogging, biking, or working out on home fitness equipment. Children are more likely to be active and stay active when they see their parents enjoying physical activity. In fact, parents who are physically active tend to have more active children (Broadwater, 2002). Steinbeck (2001) found that children of active mothers were two times more likely to have higher activity levels than children of inactive mothers, and children of active fathers were three and a half times to be more physically active than children of inactive fathers.

In all, children were six times more likely to be active when both parents were physically active. This led Steinbeck to surmise, "This is observation is likely due to learned behavior, shared environments, (and) support for activity" (p. 30). To make for a "shared environment" parents can work with their children to find physical activities they both enjoy and make plans to fulfill them daily.

Involve the whole family. Parents can make plans with the family for fun physical activity, and then make the time for it on a regular basis. The family can consider daily activities like walks after dinner, a game of bowling, a round of miniature golf, and so forth. For the weekends, the family can plan for more elaborate excursions like in the outdoors where they can hike through a local park, walk around at the zoo, or camp at a state park with a lake where they can canoe and swim. (The website for the National Park Service, http://www.nps.gov/, is a great resource to find recreational facilities in local areas). The underlying message is simple: a family that is out of the home is more likely to be engaged in physical activity than one that is confined to the home.

Restrict time dedicated to sedentary activities. Some of children's favorite pastimes – watching television, playing video games, or using computers – requires little energy, which means children burn fewer calories than when they are engaged in the more physical activities. Indeed, children today watch a lot of TV. One Nielsen report noted that children between two and 11 year-old watch about 20 hours of television per week (Brownlee, et al., 2002), and Robinson (1998) found that two to 17 year-olds spend about three years of their waking lives watching TV. Many health experts appropriately recommend that parents monitor the time children spend watching television to no more than two hours a day (Lowry, Wechsler, Galuska, Fulton, & Kann, 2002; U.S. Department of Health & Human Services, 2007b; American Academy of Pediatrics, 1995). To meet these guidelines, parents can work with their children to make some fundamental rules about how the family will spend their leisure times. Just by cutting back TV watching to an hour a day can lower the risk of obesity (Crespo, Smit, Troiano, Bartlett, Macera, & Andersen, 2001). Together, parents and children can plan for decreased time spent on sedentary activities, and commit more time to active alternatives combined with creative hobbies so that the family does not feel like all of their leisure time is spent exercising.

CONCLUSION

Parents and family play an important role in health promotion opportunities for children. If they like it or not, parents are household decision makers who directly and indirectly set the stage for their children's long-term eating and lifestyle habits. Parents can take a significant lead in enhancing their child's physical, mental, and emotional health by emphasizing correct knowledge and practices toward foods. They can provide and offer a balanced diet that is consistent with *MyPyramid* and the *Dietary Guidelines for Americans*, which means more vegetables, whole grains, low-fat and fat free dairy products, fruit, and so forth. Parents can also improve their children's health by encouraging physical activity in their daily lives. They can seek out regular, age-appropriate physical activity for the family that is fun, yet moderate or vigorous on most days of the week. All the while, parents and their children should not think of these practices as quick, temporary weight management fixes that completely cut out the foods and activities they are accustomed to and love. Instead, they should focus on adopting a healthy lifestyle where they wisely choose to restrict the foods and sedentary activities that lend themselves to the energy imbalance that leads to weight gain. When families follow these recommendations, children will build lifetime habits that enhance the body, mind and spirit.

NOTES

[i] Source: U.S. Department of Health & Human Services. (2005). *Dietary guidelines for Americans.* Retrieved March 9, 2007, from http://www.health.gov/dietaryguidelines/dga2005/document/

[ii] Source: American Heart Association. (n.d.). *How to read the new food label.* American Heart Association: Dallas, TX. Reprinted with permission.

[iii] Source: Adapted from Dairy Council of California. (2005). *Enjoy a healthy lifestyle.* Retrieved May 23, 2007, from www.mealsmatter.org. Reprinted with Permission.

[iv] Source: H.E. Butt Grocery Company. (n.d.). *Recommended snacks.* H.E. Butt Grocery Company: San Antonio, TX. Reprinted with permission.

[v] Source: American Heart Association. (2003). *Activity for life: Physical activity and fitness guide.* American Heart Association: Dallas, TX. Reprinted with Permission.

REFERENCES

American Academy of Pediatrics. (1995). Children, adolescents, and television. *Pediatrics, 96(1),* 786-787.

American Academy of Pediatrics. (2003). Policy statement: Prevention of pediatric overweight and obesity. *Pediatrics, 112(2),* 424-430.

American Dietetic Association. (1997). *Heart healthy eating for children.* The American Dietetic Association: Chicago, IL.

American Heart Association. (2007). *Exercise (physical activity) and children.* Retrieved May 27, 2007, from http://www.americanheart.org/presenter.jhtml?identifier=4596

American Obesity Association. (2007a). *Childhood obesity.* Retrieved May 28, 2007, from http://www.obesity.org/subs/childhood/prevention.shtml

American Obesity Association. (2007b). *Childhood obesity: Health risks, diagnosis and treatment.* Retrieved May 25, 2007, from http://www.obesity.org/subs/childhood/healthrisks.shtml.

Aranceta, J., Perez-Rodrigo, C., Ribas, L., & Serra-Majem, L. (2003). Sociodemographic and lifestyle determinants of food patterns in Spanish children and adolescents: The enkid study. *European Journal of Clinical Nutrition, 57(1),* 40-44.

Borzekowski, D., & Robinson, T. (2001). The 30-second effect: An experiment revealing the impact of television commercials on food preferences of preschoolers. *Journal of the American Dietetic Association, 101(1),* 42-46.

Broadwater, H. (2002). Reshaping the future for overweight kids. *RN, 65(11),* 36-42.

Brown University. (2005). *Obesity and your child: Know the facts.* The Brown University Child and Adolescent Behavior Letter. Brown University: Providence, Rhode Island.

Brownlee, S., Martens, E., McDowell, J., & Sieger, M. (2002). Too heavy, too young. *Time, 159(3),* e3.

H.E. Butt Grocery Company. (n.d.). *Spotlight on nutrition.* H.E. Butt Grocery Company: San Antonio, TX.

Cafazzo, D. (2005). *Fighting childhood obesity: A long way to go.* Retrieved May 21, 2007, from http://thenewstribune.com/news/local/v-printer/story/4634495p-4301726c.html

Chen, W. (1996). Childhood obesity: Assessment and practice. *Acta Paediatrica Sinica, 36B,* 29-31.

Crespo, C., Smit, E., Troiano, R., Bartlett, S., Macera, C., & Andersen, R. (2001). Television watching, energy intake, and obesity in US children: results from the third National Health and Nutrition Examination Survey, 1988-1994. *Archives of Pediatric Medicine, 155(3),* 360-365.

Dennison, B., Erb, T., & Jenkins, P. (2002). Television viewing and television in bedroom associated with overweight risk among low-income preschool children. *Pediatrics, 109(6),* e16.

Drohan, S. (2002). Managing early childhood obesity in the primary care setting: A behavior modification approach. *Pediatric Nursing, 28(6),* 599-610.

Fowler-Brown, A., & Kahwati, L. (2004). Prevention and treatment of overweight in children and adolescents. *American Family Physician, 69(11),* 2591-2598.

Fuhr, J., & Barclay, K. (1998). The importance of appropriate nutrition and nutrition education. *Young Children, 53(1),* 74-80.

Gable, S., & Lutz, S. (2000). Household, parent, and child contributions to childhood obesity. *Family Relations, 49(3),* 293-300.

Gassenheimer, L. (2007). *The portion plan: How to eat the foods you love & still lose weight.* DK: New York.

Gerrior, S., Putnam, J., & Bente, L. (1999). Milk and milk products: Their importance in the American diet. *Food Review, 21(2),* 29-37.

Health EDCO. (2005). *Fizzics of Soda.* Health EDCO: Waco, TX.

Hill, J. (2004). Physical activity and obesity. *The Lancet, 363(9404),* 182.

Institute of Medicine. (2004). *Industry can play a role in preventing childhood obesity.* Retrieved April 7, 2006, from http://www.iom.edu/Object.File/Master/22/613/fact%20sheet%20-%20industry%20finalBitticks.pdf.

Jacobson, M. (2007). *Liquid candy: How soft drinks are harming American's health.* Retrieved May 25, 2007, from http://www.cspinet.org/liquidcandy/.

Jain, A., Sherman, S., Chamberlin, L., Carter, Y., Power, S., & Whitaker, R. (2001). Why don't low-income mothers worry about their preschoolers being overweight? *Pediatrics, 107(5),* e17.

Lifelines. (2002). Physical activity contributes to academic success. *Vibrant Life, 18(5),* 6.

Loyo, K. (2006). *Strategic plan for the prevention of obesity in Texas: 2005-2010.* Texas Department of State Health Services: Austin, Texas.

Mandel, D. (2007). *It's not just baby fat any more.* Retrieved May 27, 2007, from http://www.keepkidshealthy.com/nutrition/not_just_baby_fat.html

McArthur, L., Anguiano, R., & Gross, M. (2004). Are household factors putting immigrant Hispanic children at risk of becoming overweight: A community-based study in Eastern North Carolina. *Journal of Community Health, 29(5),* 387-405.

Moran, R. (1999). Evaluation and treatment of childhood obesity. *American Family Physician, 59(4),* e12.

Myers, S., & Vargas, Z. (2000). Parental perceptions of the preschool obese child. *Pediatric Nursing, 26(1),* e10.

National Institute of Health. (1998). *Helping your overweight child.* Bethesda, MD: National Institute of Health.

NewsRX. (2002). *New P.E. study demonstrates vigorous exercise can lower adolescents' body fat, blood pressure.* Retrieved May 27, 2007, from http://infotrac.galegroup.com/itw/infomark/331/302/65134714w5/purl=rc1_HRCA_0_A91

Proctor, M., Moore, L., Gao, D., Cupples, L., Bradlee, M., Hood, M., & Ellison, R. (2003). Television viewing and change in body fat from preschool to early adolescence: The Framingham children's study. *International Journal of Obesity, 27(7),* 827-833.

Robinson, T. (1998). Does television cause childhood obesity? *JAMA, 279(12),* 959-960.

Smartmouth.org. (2007). *Snacktoids.* Retrieved May 25, 2007, from http://www.cspinet.org/cgi-bin/smartmouth/snacktoid.pl.

Society for Nutrition Education. (2003). Guidelines for childhood obesity prevention programs: Promoting healthy weight in children. *Healthy Weight Journal, 17(4),* 60-63.

Steinbeck, K. (2001). Obesity in children—the importance of physical activity. *Australian Journal of Nutrition and Dietetics, 58(2),* 28-32.

Tremblay, M., & Willms, J. (2003). Is the Canadian childhood obesity epidemic related to physical inactivity? *International Journal of Obesity, 27(9),* 1100-1105.

Unger, J., Reynolds, K., Shakib, S., Spruijt-Metz, D., Sun, P., & Johnson, C. (2004). Acculturation, physical activity, and fast-food consumption among Asian-American and Hispanic adolescents. *Journal of Community Health, 29(6),* 467-482.

U.S. Department of Health & Human Services. (2003). *The obesity crises in America.* Retrieved April 12, 2005, from http://www.surgeongeneral.gov/news/testimony/obesity07162003.htm.

U.S. Department of Health & Human Services. (2005). *Dietary Guideline for Americans.* Retrieved May 25, 2007, from http://www.health.gov/dietaryguidelines/dga2005/document/

U.S. Department of Health & Human Services. (2007a). *Overweight and Obesity: What You Can Do.* Retrieved May 27, 2007, from http://www.surgeongeneral.gov/topics/obesity/calltoaction/fact_whatcanyoudo.htm

U.S. Department of Health & Human Services. (2007b). *The problem of overweight in children and adolescents.* Retrieved May 27, 2007, from http://surgeongeneral.gov/topics/obesity/calltoaction/fact_adolescents.htm.

Young, L., & Nestle, M. (2002). The contribution of expanding portion sizes to the U.S. obesity epidemic. *American Journal of Public Health, 92(2),* 246-249.

Wu, F., Yu, S., Wei, I., & Yin, T. (2003). Weight-control behavior among obese children: Association with family-related factors. *Journal of Nursing Research, 11(1),* 19-28.

Zwiauer, K. (2000). Prevention and treatment of overweight and obesity in children and adolescents. *European Journal of Pediatrics, 159(1),* 56-68.

SPECIFIC HEALTH PROMOTION PROGRAMS

Thus far, the childhood obesity epidemic has been addressed from multiple perspectives from its genesis to ideas that schools and parents can use to counter the growing trend. As it stands today, many youth are making poor choices – to eat more and exercise less, which is affecting their health and well-being. If we expect health for our youth, then they must learn how to make smarter choices in their daily lives. Ergo, the obligation lies in youth-serving professionals to teach them explicitly and implicitly on how to improve their health.

Teachers, parents, and other health professionals can take an active role by helping youth understand the value of a balanced diet and regular exercise, and motivating them to make responsible decisions. Key to empowering youth lies in health promotion programs that teach concepts such as good nutrition and right amounts of physical activity, coupled with ample activities that reinforce the benefits of protected health. Well-constructed health promotion programs encompass components that develop the health-related knowledge and skills youth need to adopt lifelong attitudes, values, and behaviors that lead to a healthy lifestyle. Some of these programs are presented in this chapter. In particular, this chapters addresses:

- What are some free health programs to use at school or home?
- What are some commercially available programs?
- What are some key elements I should look for when evaluating a potential program?

WHAT ARE SOME FREE HEALTH PROGRAMS TO USE AT SCHOOL OR HOME?

The Internet is a valuable resource for finding websites that promote children's health. Many health programs, which are available on their respective homepages, offer a variety of teaching tools at no cost and can be tailored to meet children's unique needs. When making plans to address dimensions of children's health, consider the following health programs that seek to improve children's diet and physical fitness.

Active
http://www.ncpe4me.com/energizers.html

Active is a North Carolina sponsored program that promotes "Energizers," which are ten minute physical activities that teachers use in the classroom to augment academic concepts. The home page menu items offer the energizers as well as discussions on inclusive PE and PE for English Language Learners. Also available are: an invitation to the North Carolina listserve; advocacy materials; and various resources. In all, there are 22 energizers for kindergarten through second grade youngsters and 26 for the third through fifth graders, which come with tips for creating a physically active classroom. The energizers for middle school teachers are available through their respective content area links. All of the items are free; however, teachers who prefer laminated energizers can purchase them online. Table 21 is an example of a K-2 energizer.

Table 21. An Energizer from the kinder through second grade classrooms[i]

Name of Activity:	Pass It On – UNO Style
Grade Level:	1- 3
Formation:	Form a circle around perimeters of the room
Equipment:	UNO cards

Rules/Directions:
1. Teacher hands out one card to each student
2. Students identify color on card and perform activity that corresponds to that color for 10- 15 seconds:
- Blue = jump to the sky
- Red = squats
- Yellow = twists
- Green = swim

Variations:
1. Teach colors in Spanish
2. For younger children, squat and slide card on floor to the right rather than handing the card to the next person.

America on the Move (AOM)
http://aom.americaonthemove.org

This national movement encourages Americans to take simple steps to a healthier lifestyle by offering free online resources, interactive tools, and support. Children, parents, and teachers can use the "Just for Kids" link to become an AOM member and receive free program services and a personalized web page to track progress and access quizzes and puzzles. The "For Schools" link avails "Balance First" lesson plans designed for elementary youngsters (1st and 2nd, and 3rd through 5th grade) and middle school youth (6th through 8th grade). All of the lessons teach about the concept of energy balance and how to apply it in their daily lives. The six elementary "Balance First" lesson plans are comprised of learning objectives, instructional delivery information, activities, and closure statements. Corresponding worksheets follow with websites children can later visit for further information. A separate link will take site visitors to the parents' letter introducing them to "Balance First" and ways to reinforce what their children have learned at school.

The middle school curriculum includes the teacher's guide, student magazine, educator and parent letter, and classroom poster. The five lessons are comprised of learning objectives, classroom discussion and activities, environmental change activity/student challenge, home community connection, extension ideas, tips for teaching, and a list of the 2006 National Health Education Standards that align with individual lessons. Students can use the student magazine to learn about personal change, interesting nutritional facts, ways to fit in physical activity, and food labels.

Parents and older youth will find interest in the "Balance First" links. In addition to displaying the two sets of lesson plans, site visitors will notice two buttons: SMART Spot reference and counseling tools. Both of these make way to over a dozen links on the SMART Spot, which identifies food and beverage products (by their registered trademark) that meet nutritional criteria based on the FDA and National Academy of Sciences standards. Incidentally, SMART is an acronym that stands for: start with a healthy breakfast; move more; add more fruits, veggies, and whole grains; remember to hydrate; try lower calories or fat. The website mentions:

> "The Smart Spot criteria include limits for the amount of fat – including saturated and trans fat – cholesterol, sodium and added sugars. The Smart Spot designation also identifies products that are nutritious and contribute fiber, vitamins and other important nutrients, as well as products reduced in ingredients such as fat or sugar or products formulated to have specific health or wellness benefits."

The links also provide site visitors with information on food additives, allergies, and safety suggestions. The counseling tools window presents resources to help site visitors better understand food choices, portion sizes, and nutrition labels.

BAM: Body and Mind
http://www.bam.gov/

Centers for Disease Control sponsors this child-friendly website that seeks to inform site visitors about fitness, disease, and peer pressure. The home page has about 15 buttons that deal with assorted health topics that include bullying, stress, media manipulation, getting along, and so forth. The following buttons, however, deal specifically with working towards healthy behaviors:

Food & Nutrition – One of the links on this menu page is the welcome button that takes site visitors to a discussion on smart foods that lead to looking and feeling good. This link offers snack and nutritious meal ideas, and an interactive game— Dining Decisions—where players choose foods at a lunch line. They learn about the choices the made at the finale.

Physical Activity – At this link is a discussion on tracking physical activity followed by an interactive mechanism that allows site visitors to create their own activity calendar with tips on how to set goals, warm up, and plan for diverse exercises. The Activity Cards link has over two-dozen activities with directions on how to play, gear up for, and play them safely. Additionally, site visitor will find some fun facts related to each activity and icons that depict the parts of the body that are used when they engage in the physical activity. Also available is an interactive game called "I 'Heard' Hurdle" where site visitors are quizzed about physical activity rumors. Every answer that is correct allows players to proceed to the next hurdle. Lastly, site visitors can reply to a survey through the Motion Commotion link, which will use the results to identify the activities best suited for the participant.

Teacher's Corner –While the link is intended for teachers, any child or health care professional or parent can use this link to explore ways to teach children how to make healthy choices. Site visitors will find a number of interactive, educational, and fun activities under these menu items: Body Image, Energy, Epidemiology, Natural Disasters, Physical Activity, Safety, Smoking, and Stress. Separate links are found for descriptions of the lesson plan components, the reproducibles, and relevant resources.

BMI – Body Mass Index
http://www.cdc.gov/nccdphp/dnpa/bmi/index.htm

This Centers for Disease Control sponsored website is ideal for any parent or school personnel that seeks to determine the BMI of an adult or child. The homepage features two interactive BMI calculators, one for adults and one for children and adolescents, both of which allow for calculating the BMI and interpreting the results. The "About" buttons detail additional information through a series of FAQs, such as, "Why can't healthy weight ranges be provided for children and teens?" And, "My two children have the same BMI values, but one is considered overweight and the other is not. Why is that?"

CANFIT
http://www.canfit.org/

The CANFIT campaign is designed specifically for California's low income, ethnic 10- to 14-year-old youth. The homepage consists of many menu items that site visitors will find resourceful such as the "Nutrition and Fitness" links that have many worksheets that can be downloaded and used in the classroom or at home.

The Nutrition link offers site visitors a number of resources: healthy eating tips for after school programs; nutrition activities like how to conduct a taste test, help youth make better snack choices, and encourage youth to create their own health campaigns; and an actual healthy snack plan that spells out the specific snacks that children can enjoy on specific days of the week. Another button allows site visitors to download a one-page handout that teaches how advertising lures people to consume food products. The "Nutrition and Activities Matter" link leads to a two-page activity that reinforces the common consequences of eating behaviors. Following is a seven-page guide for a lesson called "What are you really paying for?" The lesson invites youth to explore how much money they spend on convenience foods and then work out ways to reduce some of the costs. Two more handouts are found on the link: a lesson on food labels where youth search food products and fill in a blank label, and tips on applying the *Dietary Guidelines for Americans* for after-school programs. At the "Fitness" link site visitors will find the physical activity pyramid that describes the amount of physical activity children need and ideas for working individually, with groups and with parents. There are other links that take site visitors to prior newsletters that offer ideas for incorporating physical activity in the classroom.

Eat Smart. Play Hard.
http://www.fns.usda.gov/eatsmartplayhard/

This USDA Food and Nutrition Service website has assorted resources divided for three kinds of consumers: children, their parents, and health professionals. Child site visitors can make their way to a cyberspace village comprised of ten store-like buildings, that each lead to categorized information. The respective buttons are:

Town Library – By way of this button, site visitors can retrieve six types of materials. *Power Panther Tales*, which are comics about the program mascot and his sidekick Slurp who teach children to eat healthy and be physically active. Another link is clip art of Power Panther and Slurp that can be downloaded in color, black and white, or half tones. The Activity Sheets link is comprised of four one-page handouts (three are in Spanish) where students use their knowledge of healthy habits to complete the written exercises. Two of the handouts are "seek-and-find" games, while the remaining is a coloring sheet of the MyPyramid for Kids. The "Activity & Sticker Book for Kids Ages 6 to 8" link takes children to a 13-page booklet of puzzles. A letter to parents prefaces the story about Power Panther and Slurp, and concludes with tips on how to use the booklet. The Food Experiment link offers visitors access to six experiments ranging from separating milk into curds and whey to testing foods for their fat content. The "MyPyramid for Kids" link takes visitors to three levels of lesson plans on the food guidance system. Each level is comprised of the teacher's guide and reproducible worksheets. School personnel can order hard copies of the instructional material, which will include a CD of MyPyramid Blast Off game, Power Panther songs, Go Fish card games, a poster, and tips for families. The last link is the Other Fun Stuff, which allows site visitors to download a MyPyramid for Kids poster and two MyPyramid for Kids worksheets.

Theatre – This link lets site visitors view three multi-media messages: one is the unveiling of Power Panther; the other is PowerPoint slide of the Power Up Moves dance that children can mirror; and the third is Power Panther dancing.

Post Office – Here, site visitors can download seven e-cards for various occasions and send them to friends or family members.

Eat Smart Grill – The link opens a window to various healthy recipes that are divided into three categories: fruity favorites, snacks, and sandwiches. The recipes are simple and diagrams show Power Panther following the steps for preparation. Each recipe has an accompanying worksheet for children to complete.

Fun Times Arcade – This link offers interactive games by way of three buttons: Games, MyPyramid Blast Off Game, and Links to Other Fun Stuff. In the Games window, children can play: Gardening Game (where users try to fend of weeds and insects from their garden); Power Panther Maze (where users help Power Panther make his way to a bowl of fruit); "Eat Smart. Play Hard. Word Jumble" (where users unscramble health-related vocabulary); and Power Panther's Art Room (where users can create and print a picture using provided icons). The object of the MyPyramid Blast Off Game is to prepare for a space trip by choosing foods and physical activity that fuel the user's rocket for long lasting travel. When users choose the wrong foods and sedentary activities, the rocket does not travel far; when the foods that meet the MyPyramid guidelines and at least 60 minutes of physical activity are chosen, the rocket will travel in space. The "Links to Other Fun Stuff" gives access to assorted games, quizzes, and puzzles.

Travel – Through this link is a window of an informative slide ("Where in the States is Power Panther?" where children learn interesting facts about the 50 states), two reproducibles (that are profiles that children fill out with interesting information about themselves), and a treasure hunt worksheet that instructs children to look for specific healthy items at the grocery store.

Farmers' Market – Some of the resources found on this window are found elsewhere, but there are two worksheets (one to make a food diary and another to plan for healthier eating), and a link to the Farm Service Agency's website for children, which offers an array of resources including an interactive game called Agventure.

Playground – The link offers site visitors ideas for spending their time engaged in physical activity. The link "Let's Go Fly a Kite!" teaches how to make a kite and describes the conditions best for kite flying. The "Explore Your Community" link encourages visitors to hunt in their community for as many items on a prescribed list. The "Activity Games" link lists physical activity games that children can play. The games are divided into five sections: pretend games and imagination; rhythmic and balance games; running and jumping games; throwing, kicking, and catching games; and tumbling, rolling, crawling, and climbing games.

The link for the parents' division is comprehensive as it is designed to help them become role models for children. The main buttons make way to information and resources to help parents get started on their path toward a healthy lifestyle. These include:

Getting Ready – This link takes visitors to a tracking card that site visitors can download to track all the foods that are consumed and the amount of physical activity they engage in a given day. The card helps users monitor progress, stay motivated, and celebrate successes. The other window, Staying with the Lifestyle, offers pointers for daily living that includes ideas like setting realistic goals.

Making Smart Choices – Here, four links discuss ways to overcome the obstacles in life that make it difficult to become healthy. One of the links is a tutorial on MyPyramid, while the other three offer ideas for getting started on a healthier lifestyle. The ideas range from categories like ordering at a fast food restaurant to shopping at the grocery store.

Make It Quick and Easy – Healthful recipes for salads, entrees, side dishes, and desserts can be found at this link as well as a two-week menu starter and tips for menu planning.

Play Hard Your Way – This link starts with a discussion of the benefits on physical activity and follows with ideas for engaging in physical activity at home, work, and play. An additional link offers helpful advice to overcome some of the challenges that stand in the way of physical activity.

Tools to Help You – As the title indicates, the link here provides some simple resources to help site visitors maintain a healthy lifestyle. These include: a seven-day menu planner; a calorie burning chart that shows the number of calories that are burned in 30 and 60 minutes for moderate and vigorous physical activities; and a link to the MyPyramid website so that visitors can customize a food guide with respect to their age, gender, and level of physical activity.

While health or school professionals can certainly use the resources for children and parents, they too have their own special link to a broad range of materials. Some of the materials are repeated here, but the most useful link for the professional is the "Eat Smart. Play Hard. Collection." Site visitors will find Power Panther showcasing a file cabinet with file drawers that are button links. The file "Professional Tools" affords site visitors worksheets that can be downloaded so that children can make a Power Panther costume. Another file drawer is called Power Pac, which avails an array of documents to successfully implement the campaign in a school or a community setting through four links: Introduction, About the Spokesperson, Promotional and Educational Materials, Publicity Information.

Fruits and Veggies – More Matters
http://www.fruitsandveggiesmatter.gov/

This simple, interactive website supports the "Fruits and Veggies – More Matters" initiative, which encourages more fruit and vegetables consumption. One web button will create an individualized regimen after visitors type in their age, gender, and amount of physical activity that is exerted daily to determine how much fruit and vegetables should be eaten every day. Another website button introduces a fruit or vegetable each month, and follows with its nutritional information. The last two buttons are meal preparation specific. One button accesses a database of healthy recipes that can be searched with key words, while the other recommends ways to fill the day with fruit and vegetables. Publications can be downloaded by way of the index panel, some of which include:

- How many fruits and vegetables do you need? (Available in Spanish)
- Three simple steps to eating more fruits and vegetables (Available in Spanish)
- Choose Smart, Choose Health
- Why do Fruits and Vegetables Matter to Men?
- How to Use Fruits and Vegetables to Help Manage Your Weight (Available in Spanish)
- Can Eating Fruits and Vegetables Help People to Manage their Weight? Research into Practice No. 1

Get Fit!
http://www.presidentschallenge.org/pdf/getfit.pdf

This handbook for youth (for ages six through 17) is a publication of the President's Council on Physical Fitness and Sports and is intended to help youth get active and in shape to meet the President's fitness challenge. The 32-pages are filled with encouraging messages on ways to improve children's current and future health as well as motivate them through the presidential awards program. The curriculum begins with an explanation of two overarching acronyms designed to enhance their fitness level: SMART (Specific, Measurable, Action Oriented, Realistic, Timely) and FITT (Frequency, Intensity, Type, Time). A discussion ensues over the importance of warming up and includes nearly a dozen warm-up exercises coupled with photos on how to perform them correctly. Also included in the handbook are a series of muscular strength and endurance exercises with photos and a BMI calculator.

Jump Up & Go!
http://www.bluecrossma.com/common/en_US/index.jsp

"Jump Up & Go!" is a Blue Cross Blue Shield of Massachusetts sponsored health initiative designed to help children and adults become physically active and develop lifetime healthy habits. The program advocates a "5-2-1" message that promotes eating five fruit and vegetables a day; limiting TV and media use to two hours per day; and engaging in at least one hour of physical activity each day. There are three links to access the respective resources:

Parents – This link discusses why parents must guide their children to a healthy lifestyle and leads to a "kit" of items to help them get started. The tools include: a survey on their children's school for parents to complete to help them advocate for healthier schools; a weekly log sheet to track the "5-2-1" progress; a bank of family friendly recipes; tips for daily walking; an eight-page brochure on the "5-2-1" message and assorted tips on what parents can do support a healthy lifestyle; a question and answer handout; nutrition tips for eating smart; activity tips for getting fit; and a list of web-based resources.

Teachers – The link includes a discussion on why teachers matter in the childhood obesity crises. The resources in the teachers' kit can be used in the $4^{th} - 8^{th}$ grade classroom or through an after school program. Some of the resources here include: a handout on what teachers should know about youth, nutrition, and physical activity; tips for promoting "Jump Up & Go!" in the classroom; fun and interactive games to reinforce the '5-2-1'" message; ideas for the larger school community; a one-page question and answer brochure for teachers; and a campaign poster.

Clinicians – Resources here are designed for clinicians to use with their patients. The web page acknowledges, "The office visit gives you an excellent opportunity to screen and classify BMI, counsel families on the importance of healthy eating and active living, and when needed, coordinate participation in school and community based nutrition and physical activity programs. Your message can be as simple as "5-2-1." Some of the toolkit resources available through this link are: BMI growth charts for boys and girls; a nutrition and physical activity fact sheet; a physical activity and nutrition survey that patients can complete while they wait to see the doctor; "Are You A Healthy Kid?" brochure that can be distributed at the doctor's office; and a presentation on helping the clinician better understand the CDC 2000 Growth Charts.

Kidnetic.com
http://www.kidnetic.com/

Kidnetic.com is an interactive website that challenges youth to develop their fitness, eat healthier, learn about body organs, and read the answers to most frequently asked questions about health. The Kore button – subtitled Move –

offers site visitors a range of indoor and outdoor games. Site visitors will enjoy playing three of the Kore games because they are inviting. Scavenger Hunt, for instance, asks users to retrieve household items as fast they can while the website times them. A stopwatch also times site visitors when they take the fitness challenge, which asks visitors to complete some indoor exercises. The Move Mixer is just as engaging because it allows youth to string dance movements into one continuous dance that a cyber mechanical man and the site visitor can then dance to.

Site visitors will also find about 70 recipes in the Recipe Roundup section. These can be retrieved through eight buttons: Family Friendly, Breakfast Bonanza, Brown Bag Specials, Gross Out Delights, Featured, Super Sides, Smart Snacks, and Dinner Winners. In addition to the general directions for preparation, the recipes also list the nutritional value of the recommended servings.

The "Inner G" button makes way to a game where site visitors click and drag vital organs to their proper place on a skeletal body found on the web page. When the answer is correct, a prompt appears to inform the visitor of the foods that are most beneficial for the respective organ. Immediately following are recipes of foods that serve the organ well with added links for further research. The last button is titled "Bright Papers: Read All About It!", which provides a range of discussions on topics germane to health. The topics (and tips) are divided into six categories: Featured (e.g., "Should Kids Go on a Diet to Lose Weight"), Fitness (e.g., "Five Fun Ways to Get Physical"), Food (e.g., "Are You Snack Smart?"), Fun (e.g., "Be a Food Ad Detective"), Feelings (e.g., "Self-Esteem and You"), and For Parents (e.g., "For Steps for Helping an Overweight Child").

KidsHealth for Kids
http://kidshealth.org/index.html

The Nemours Foundation sponsors this program. At this home site, there are three separate buttons for parents, children, and teens. The "parents" button offers practical parenting information and news on assorted topics ranging from children's emotions and behavior to positive parenting. A click of the "Nutrition & Fitness" button will retrieve information on eating, diet, exercise, and so forth as it relates to children. A number of resources here can help parents keep their children healthy with the right doze of foods and exercises. See Table 22.

The "kids" site is just as enterprising with over a dozen links that deal with topics germane to the body. Site visitors interested in health issues as they relate to diet and exercise will find two buttons particularly useful: Staying Healthy and Recipes. A click of the Staying Healthy button makes way to over 70 links that are divided into four categories: Keeping Fit and Having Fun; Being Good to My Body; Fabulous Food; and Wondering Weight. Site visitors can learn a great deal about foods and meal preparation from a wide range of recipes, including some specifically for children who are vegetarians or lactose intolerant or those who live with Cystic Fibrosis, diabetes, and Celiac Disease. Adolescents will find answers, advice, and straight talk at the "teen" link. There are over 100 links found in the

Table 22. The many topics found at the Nutrition & Fitness link of the Kids Health parents segment[ii]

Fitness & Exercise

Bike Safety
Cold Weather Sports & Your Family
Compulsive Exercise
Do You Know How to Feed Your Child Athlete?
Exercising During Pregnancy
Fitness and Youth 13- to 18-Year-Old
Fitness and Youth 2- to 3-Year-Old
Fitness and Youth 4- to 5-Year-Old
Fitness and Youth 6- to 12-Year-Old

Fitness for Kids Who Don't Like Sports
Kids and Exercise
Osgood-Schlatter Disease
Preventing Children's Sports Injuries
Raising a Fit Preschooler
Signing Kids Up for Sports
Sportsmanship
Steroids
Strength Training and Your Child

Nutrition & Weight

Binge Eating Disorder
Body Mass Index Charts
Breakfast Basics
Breastfeeding vs. Formula Feeding
Caffeine and Your Child
Calcium and Your Child
Carboyhdrates, Sugar, and Your Child
Cholesterol and Your Child
Cystic Fibrosis and Nutrition
Deciphering Food Labels
Do You Know How to Feed Your Child Athlete?
Eating Disorders
Eating During Pregnancy
Egg Allergy
Egg Allergy Diet
Failure to Thrive
Fats and Your Child
Feeding Your 1- to 2-Year-Old
Feeding Your 1- to 3-Month-Old

Feeding Your 4- to 7-Month-Old
Feeding Your 8- to 12-Month-Old
Feeding Your Newborn
Fiber and Your Child
Food Allergies
Food Safety for Your Family
Healthy Eating
Hunger and Malnutrition
Iron and Your Child
Keeping Portions Under Control
Milk Allergy Diet
Nut and Peanut Allergy
Nut and Peanut Allergy Diet
Overweight and Obesity
Pica
School Lunches
The Food Guide Pyramid
Vegetarianism
Your Child's Weight

Nutrition & Fitness Q&As

Can Too Much Juice Discolor Teeth?
Does Skim Milk Provide the Same Nutrients as Whole Milk?
How Can I Calculate Calories From Fat?
How Can I Get My Child to Eat Vegetables?
How Much Exercising Is Too Much?
How Should I Deal With a Picky Eater?
Is Caffeinated Soda OK for Kids?
My Child May Have an Eating Disorder — What Can I Do?
Should I Start My Child on an Exercise Program?

What Are the Symptoms of an Overeating Disorder?
What Can I Do for a Child With an Eating Disorder?
When Can a Young Child Start Exercising?
When Should My Child Switch to Skim Milk?
Why Does My Toddler Eat Dog Food?
Why Is Breakfast So Important?

Food & Fitness button, which are divided into nine areas: Total Well-being; Sports Journal; Dieting; Nutrition Basics; Exercise; Sports; Problems with Food & Exercise; Food & Fitness Q&As.

Learn to be Healthy
http://www.learntobehealthy.org/

The Highmark Foundation sponsors this Pennsylvania-based initiative on good nutrition for children and seeks to develop innovative, high quality, effective health education programs as part of a greater plan to address the childhood obesity epidemic. Site visitors register with Learn to be Healthy to access a wide range health-based lesson plans and web-based activities. Germane to the topic are two links: Eating Healthy for second, third, and fourth grade youngsters, and Nutrition and Physical Activities for fourth through sixth graders.

The *Eating Healthy* link is comprised of ten curriculum modules called e-learning kits, which are comprised of lesson plans on "Fueling my special body" with answer keys and web-based games that students can play to reinforce the connections between the digestive system, the food pyramid, and the benefits of good nutrition. Following is a second set of lesson plans specific to the health benefits of dairy products. The window from *Nutrition and Physical Activities* link also leads to ten e-learning kits on food and fitness with pre- and post-tests. The lessons are similar to the ones designed for the younger students; however, these include a culminating event where students work their way to the track and field.

Portion Distortion
http://hp2010.nhlbihin.net/portion/

The National Institute of Health offers this insightful, interactive website that allows visitors to think about portion control. Two of the buttons quiz visitors on how portion sizes (in terms of calories) have grown in 20 years and follow with what it takes to burn off the extra calories. The button "Keep an Eye on Portion Size" discusses the difference between portions and servings, and offers a serving size card (using common objects as standards) that can be downloaded and used for meal planning. Another button will take site visitors to the American Dietetic Association's Food Exchange List where visitors can locate foods – ranging from very lean proteins to starches – and their serving sizes that can be substituted within each group. A unique feature of the site is the menu planner, which visitors can use to create a meal or add up daily calorie consumption.

Shape It Up
http://www.horizon-bcbsnj.com/shapeitup/index.asp

Shape It Up is an obesity intervention program created jointly by Horizon Blue Cross Blue Shield of New Jersey and Rutgers University's School of Pharmacy. The program teaches elementary-age youngsters about physical activity, healthy eating, and the risks associated with obesity. Certified teachers created all of the materials and accompanying lesson plans so that they are developmentally appropriate and meet the New Jersey State health standards. The Shape It Up homepage has four buttons that parents, youth, and school personnel will find particularly useful as they offer concrete steps to help children become and stay healthy. These are:

Healthy Eating Tips: This button retrieves a family guide that helps parents and their children cultivate healthier eating and exercise habits. A discussion ensues over how families can make lifestyle changes with assorted tips found in six avenues: family meals; stocking up on health foods; being a role model; helping children help themselves; keeping tabs on children's weight; and children, sports and exercise.

Target Heart Rate for Children: This button presents a table of ideal heart rates for children. Site visitors can find a child's age group and the corresponding target heart rates for resting, average, and exercising, and then work accordingly toward a specific goal.

Health Food Chart: Here site visitors will find a chart divided into five primary colors of fruit and vegetables. Fruit and vegetables are listed categorically accompanied with specific health benefits of each (e.g. fights cancer, improves vision, helps memory, etc), which helps visitors understand why it is important to vary fruits and vegetables consumption throughout the day.

Program Materials: The reproducible handouts Food Pyramid, Activity Book and Family Guide, and a Healthy Food Journal can be downloaded from this button. The Food Pyramid is a one-page flyer that details the number of servings from each food group that should be consumed daily. Two additional information boxes offer tips on meeting the recommended servings and incorporating physical activity every day. The activity booklet is an eight-page document filled with ways to enhance a well-balanced diet and become a fit child. Graphic organizers are provided so that the children can reflect on their current lifestyle and plan for an improved life. Children can use the "My Healthy Days Journal" to keep track of their daily consumption and degree of exercise.

VERB ™ *It's what you do.*
http://www.cdc.gov/youthcampaign/

In June 2002, the Centers for Disease Control launched the national youth media campaign known as VERB. The campaign uses commercial advertising to encourage youth between the ages of nine to 13 to engage in physical activity every day. The VERB message grew from physical activities youth could try to one where they explore physical activity through different VERB actions. VERB now publicizes that physical activity can be easily accomplished every day by varying means. Most of the communication is delivered by way of network TV public service announcements during times when youth are likely watching, but the VERB message can be seen on billboards, city buses, movie theatres, on the Internet, and heard on the radio; assorted publications are also available. A component of the campaign is targeted toward ethnic audiences and is advertised in different languages. Campaign personnel also distribute physical activity information at cultural and heritage festivals.

There are many free resources for adults on the VERB website including:

1) Colorful brochures designed to inspire families to play together (60: Play. Every Day. Any Way; Active Children. Active, Active Families: A Helpful Guide to Parents; Healthy Kids, Healthy Families);

2) One-page handouts of tips to make physical activity a part of children's daily lives (Tips for Teachers, Tips for Parents, Tips for Organizations); and

3) Brochures for school personnel to lead students toward physical activity (You Inspire Strong Minds; They Will Follow Your Lead).

A special button on the VERB website allows youth to access materials designed especially for them. Some of the resources include:

- VERB Yellowball – includes five "Activity Action" cards that youth can follow to get moving. One of the cards, for instance, invites youth to make and participate in an obstacle course.

- VERB Make It UP – has assorted games that have been modified from the traditional way of playing. For instance, Hip Hop Scotch is adapted so that whenever the tossed rock lands on a square, youth make a specific rhythm and dance movement.

- VERB Crossover – these are games that are components of one sport mixed with another. For instance, Dribbleball is a game of basketball crossed with soccer where the students use their feet to dribble the ball. As they approach the basket they can grab the ball and shoot for the hoop.

- VERB Play without Borders – Here students explore games played around the world and create new ways to play them.

- Anytime Double Time – Like VERB Crossover, youth take elements from one sport and combine them with another to make their own game.

- VERB Appreciation Day – Youth select a physical activity that could be celebrated for an entire day. The activity can be one where the students learn a new form of exercise like Yoga, Ultimate Frisbee, or Hip Hop Dance, or engage in familiar activities like biking, hula "hoping" or hiking.

- Student Planner – This weekly planner inspires youth to engage in a new VERB each week.

Weight-control Information Network
http://win.niddk.nih.gov/publications/index.htm

The Weight-control Information Network (WIN) is the initiative of the National Institute of Diabetes and Digestive and Kidney Diseases. This information service disseminates assorted scientific-based resources on weight control, obesity, physical activity, and related nutritional issues. There are four main buttons to access the information. One of the buttons gives way to over 25 free publications, which can be downloaded or requested by mail. While a number of the publications are intended for adults (e.g., "Fit and Fabulous as You Mature"), some are child- and adolescent-based that can be tailored to meet the needs of youth. These publications include:

- *Active at Any Size* shows how any person regardless of their weight status can engage in physical activity. The publication begins with a discussion on the benefits of exercising, addresses ways to get to started, overcome common barriers, and outlines some tips for what works.
- *Celebrate the Beauty of Youth* is a two-page brochure of tips for moving more and eating better.
- *Helping Your Child: Tips for Parents* informs parents on to help their children become healthier. The content focuses on what children should eat including a discourse on source of nutrition and healthy snack ideas. The latter part of the booklet discusses physical activity and how parents can help their children become more physically fit. A list of resources concludes the document.
- *Energize Yourself and Your Family* seeks to encourage parents to improve their family's health through movement and eating well. In addition to a number of tips to arrive at a healthy lifestyle is a tutorial on food labels and portion control.
- *Helping Your Overweight Child* is a four-page pamphlet that describes how parents can support and encourage overweight children. Assorted tips are categorized into two areas: healthy eating habits and daily physical activity. A list of resources trails behind the outlines of suggestions.
- *Just Enough For You: About Food Portions* is a comprehensive publication devoted to portion control. Readers can learn about the difference between portions and servings, how to use household items as standard for portions, and how to control portions when eating in and outside of the home.
- *Walking....A Step in the Right Direction* is a two-page brochure packed with suggestions related to walking as an exercise. Immediately following a discussion on why walking is good exercise are ideas for stretching, how to start a walking program, safety tips, and a sample walking program.

WHAT ARE SOME COMMERCIALLY AVAILABLE PROGRAMS?

There are a number of books available at Gopher (www.gophersport.com) and PE central (http://www.pecentral.org) that offer lesson plans and tips on physical activity like games, fitness, developing sport-specific skills, and other health-related instruction. See Table 24 for a list of titles. However, schools or child-serving organizations that would like to purchase health promotion programs with lesson plans and an elaborate curriculum may find these programs worthwhile.

Table 23. Some books and curricula titles devoted to physical activity and health related topics available through Gopher and PE Central

Gopher
www.gophersport.com

101 Fun Warm-Up and Cool Down Games	Fun and Games Book
Best New Games	Games to Keep Kids Moving
Celebration Games	Healthy Hearts in the Zone
Character Education: 43 Fitness	Ready to Use PE Activities
Activities for Community Building	Thinking on Your Feet
Dynamic Physical Education for	The Ultimate Playground and Recess
Secondary School Students	Game Book
Essentials of Team Building	

PE Central
www.pecentral.org

40 Years in the Gym-Favorite	Life Skills Health Activities Book
Physical Education Activities	No Gym? No Problem! Limited
85 Engaging Movement Activities	Space Activities
(K-6)	No Standing Around in My Gym
bSAFE, bFIT! Program for kids: A	No Props: Great Games with No
Physical Activity & Nutrition	Equipment
Program	PE2theMax: Maximize Skills,
Classroom Jeopardy Game	Participation, Teamwork & Fun
Creating Healthy Habits: An	Physical Education Funbook for
Adventure Guide to Teaching Health	Grades K-8
and Wellness	Planet Health: An Interdisciplinary
The Elementary Physical Education	Curriculum for Teaching MS School
Workbook	Nutrition
Fit Kids: Classroom Workout DVD	Tools for Teaching Health
Healthy Eating & Exercise: CD Rom	
(PreK-Elem)	

1% or Less Campaign
http://www.cspinet.org/nutrition/1less.htm

The Center for Science in the Public Interest (CSPI) publishes this health education campaign that seeks to motivate adults and children over the age of two to switch from whole or 2% milk to 1% or fat-free (skim) milk. The website mentions, "The campaign focuses on milk because of its important contribution to both health and disease. Milk is an important source of calcium and vitamin D for strong bones. However, whole and 2% milk also are among the biggest contributors of saturated fat to Americans' diets. Switching to 1% or skim milk is one of the easiest ways for Americans to get the calcium they need, while reducing their saturated-fat intake and heart-disease risk." As it stands today two out of three children who drink milk at school choose 2% or whole milk.

The School Kit contains fact sheets, instructional activity worksheets, visual displays about the amount of fat in milk, and information on how to plan and implement the campaign. Also included are: strategies for marketing low-fat and skim milk to students; signs to hang around the cafeteria encouraging students to choose low-fat and skim milk; directions on how to conduct milk taste tests; ideas for using peer education; and handouts for parents. A number of health experts endorse the campaign. Basil Rifkind, M.D., for instance, of the National Institute of Health writes, "The campaign seems to have been a simple, successful, and relatively inexpensive undertaking to reduce one of the major sources of saturated fat. Milk is a healthy drink provided that the fat is removed. This approach has the potential to save many lives." The School Kit is available through the website for $15.

California Adolescent Nutrition and Fitness Program (CANFit)
http://www.canfit.org/pdf/CANFit%20Super%20Manual.pdf
http://www.canfit.org/phat/order.html

Two CANFit resources can be purchased through the respective websites. The first is titled, *CANFit Super Manual* and is marketed as an all-in-one resource ideal for youth service providers looking to promote nutrition education and physical activity into daily programming. The *Super Manual* is 135 pages of lesson plans, handouts, evaluation tips, and recipes, and guides users with program ideas, assessment, and curriculum standards. The cost is $40, which includes a colorful binder ($35 without).

The second resource is called *Promoting Health Activities Together* or *PHAT*. This is a community-based campaign targeted to improve the nutrition and physical activity lifestyle of 10- to 14-year-old African Americans who live in the San Francisco Bay area. The program has a hip-hop element that is evident in the nutrition and fitness raps, artwork, and dance routines found in the multi-media package. It includes: a 55-minute video on nutrition and physical activity and a 40-minute tutorial on hip-hop dance routines; a CD compilation of original hip-hop music with a 10-minute workout mix; and a 36-page guide on how to enhance programming. *PHAT* organizers maintain that the program is effective. The website mentions, "Results from the surveys taken one year after the completion of the P.H.A.T. campaign show that many of the youth maintained knowledge and positive attitudes, but the decreases in the percentage of youth drinking less soda and more water show that in order to maintain positive behaviors, healthy messages must be reinforced on a regular basis." The package is available for $100. Organizations that work with low-income youth can purchase it for $55.

Coordinated Approach to Child Health in Texas (CATCH)
http://www.sph.uth.tmc.edu/catch/

CATCH seeks to produce healthy children and school environments. Specifically, it is a comprehensive school-based health program that is designed to improve elementary-aged children's fitness by increasing their level of physical activity and healthy food choices by promoting healthy eating habits. Studies using scientific methods suggest that CATCH works to change behaviors that last well into adulthood. Research published in *Journal of the American Medical Association* (1996) and *Archives of Pediatric & Adolescent Medicine* (1999) found that CATCH participants:
1. reduced total fat and saturated fat content of school lunches;
2. increased moderate-to-vigorous physical activity during P.E. classes; and
3. improved students' self-reported eating and physical activity behaviors.
CATCH has four program components: the "Go For Health" classroom curriculum; the nutrition aspect titled "Eat Smart"; CATCH PE; and the "Home Team" family program.

"Go For Health" is about teaching students healthy habits. According to the website, "CATCH Go For Health is based on Social Learning Theory which targets changes in specific environmental, personality and behavioral factors that influence children's health behavior. A sequential storyline throughout the curricula revolves around a group of cartoon characters, *Hearty Heart and Friends*. The characters teach students about necessary eating, physical activity and non-tobacco use habits which promote health." The sequence of lesson plans include: Jump Into Health where students learn about "everyday" and "sometimes" foods (sic); Everyday Foods for Everyday Health, which is a reinforcement of the concepts learned in the kindergarten curriculum; Celebrate Health that teaches children to identify hidden fats in foods; Hearty Heart & Friends, which targets change in children's behavior; Taking Off introduces the concept of "Go" (go for foods that contain the lowest amount of fat), "Slow" (eat foods that are higher in fats less often), and "Whoa" (eat the foods highest in fat less often than GO or SLOW foods); Breaking through Barriers where students learn to overcome common barriers to a healthy lifestyle.

The CATCH curriculum is comprised of:
*   Lesson plans that can be taught independent of the others or to supplement the content areas such as math, reading, writing, and so forth;
*   Guides, reproducibles, transparency masters, and suggestions for role-playing, hands-on activities, and positive reinforcement;
*   References on background information on key topics.
CATCH PE is a developmentally appropriate physical education program that teaches fitness, skill competency, and the importance of physical activity in everyday life. CATCH PE: provides meaningful experiences; increases the moderate-to-vigorous physical activity in PE; promotes adequate amounts of

physical activity throughout life; and engages the students in fun and motivating activities. Schools can purchase three PE kits: Kinder – Second Grade, 3rd – 5th Grade, and 6th – 8th grades.

"Eat Smart" uses the school cafeteria as an extension of the curriculum so that students can practice the concept of "Go, Slow, and Whoa." There are four target areas, known as the 4 P's, so that cafeteria services can transform the school cafeteria into a nutritional environment. *Planning* considers creating nutritious meals for children. In this vein, the cafeteria service workers can look to "Eat Smart" for suggestions on recipes that meet the School Meal Initiative goals. *Purchasing* works to help connect the service workers with venders that supply food options that meet the criteria for fat and saturated fat. *Preparation/Production* teaches service workers techniques that lower the fat and saturated fat in meals that children consume at school. Lastly, *Promotion* is a tool that the service workers can use to enliven the cafeteria by way of marketing suggestions.

The "Home Team" is the family component of the curriculum where parents and the family are motivated to change their behavior as well. Some of the Home Team objectives are to: provide opportunities for parents and family members to visit the school and participate in CATCH; influence changes in the home environment that reflect the changes that are happening at school; and get the families involved as much as possible. To work toward these goals there are activity booklets that children take home and complete with their parents. This component also comes with suggestions for family fun nights where parents, community members, school personnel, and children come together to engage in fun, interactive, and high-energy activities.

Flaghouse, Inc. publishes CATCH materials. See http://www.flaghouse.com/CatchPE.asp for price details.

Eat Well & Keep Moving - An Interdisciplinary Curriculum for Teaching Upper Elementary School Nutrition and Physical Activity
http://www.humankinetics.com/products/showproduct.cfm?isbn=0736030964

This curriculum seeks to improve the nutrition and physical activity levels of upper grade elementary school students by teaching them to eat better and stay active. The interdisciplinary, skills-building approach began as a Harvard School of Public Health and Baltimore Public Schools research project and has won awards for excellence from the United States Department of Agriculture's Promising Practice Award (1997), and the Dannon Institute Award for Excellence in Community Nutrition (2000). Extensive field tests suggest that the curriculum is effective because participants ate more fruit and vegetables, reduced their consumption of saturated and total fats, watched less television, and improved their nutrition and physical activity knowledge.

Eat Well & Keep Moving is comprehensive. The website reports:

"This complete resource includes everything you need to teach students about nutrition and fitness in a classroom setting or to launch an effective schoolwide program. The ready-to-use materials fit easily into any existing curriculum: These materials help classroom teachers overcome any uneasiness they may have about presenting unfamiliar health topics while they build students' language arts, math, science, social studies, and physical education skills."

The program includes: 44 lesson plans; a CD-ROM of lessons, units, worksheets, and instructional ideas; fun and engaging school-wide campaigns; and reproducibles. The curriculum is distributed by Human Kinetics and costs $47.

Healthy Start
Animal Trackers
Healthy Hops
http://www.healthy-start.com/

The Healthy Start Company has programs devoted to pre-school nutrition and physical activity for the sake of promoting healthy behaviors. Their website contends, "Our programs are created by a team of the best and the brightest in the fields of obesity prevention, nutrition, physical activity, and educational content. These timely and exemplary programs are extensively researched, evaluated and published in over 20 professional journals. The programs are designed to be engaging and fun for young children with stories, games, songs and rhymes. They are adaptable to a variety of preschool environments and easy to integrate into any early childhood education curriculum." To prevent childhood obesity, the company seeks to help children develop a healthy lifestyle by teaching them about:

- Making positive, healthy lifestyle choices now and through their lifetime;
- Healthy eating and physical activity behaviors;
- Concepts and skills to prevent obesity later in life;
- Self-esteem and how to maintain a healthy one; and
- The damaging affects of tobacco, alcohol, and other drugs.

These objectives are carried out in three separate curricula for children between the ages of three to five.

The first is titled, *Healthy Start* ($179), which can be used to teach wellness concepts and behaviors. The program is comprised of 12 instructional units that are focused on the child, environment, and the family and incorporate stories, songs, rhymes, art projects, and activities. Some of the concepts include: Eating for Health; Enjoying Active Play Every Day; Getting Along with Others; Feeling Good About Me; Safety and Care of the Body; Saying No to Drugs and Smoking; Taking Care of the Environment; and Staying Safe in the Sun. Recordings of songs and poems reinforcing health concepts, 12 colorful posters, and take home activities for the family to complete are part of the *Healthy Start* package.

Animal Trackers ($79.95) deals with physical activity and motor skills where children learn and practice gross motor skills like catching a ball, running, kicking, jumping, hoping, and so forth. The program includes ten units on motor skill development, each with a different animal theme, and over 60 classroom activities, a music CD, a poster set, and 10 take home family activities. *Healthy Hop* ($39.95) reinforces the concept of "healthy eating, healthy play," where children learn about the body and vital organ functions and the foods that keeps them in optimal shape. The program includes over 25 classroom activities covering nutrition and physical activity, seven reproducibles linked to classroom lessons, and take home activities. The Healthy Start homepage has a menu of links that will take site visitors to ordering information as well as sample pages from each curriculum.

SPARK
http://www.sparkpe.org/

SPARK prides itself in being the "new" PE because it is more active, inclusive, and fun. SPARK started out as a research program that received funding from the National Institute of Health and evolved into an elementary physical education program that seeks to advance the quantity and quality of physical activity in children's daily lives. According to their website, "SPARK strives to improve the health of children and adolescents by disseminating evidence-based physical activity and nutrition programs that provide curriculum, staff development, follow-up support, and equipment to teachers of Pre-K through 12th grade students. SPARK strives to achieve outstanding customer satisfaction through timely delivery and exceptional service." The SPARK objectives are to help children: develop and maintain acceptable levels of physical fitness; develop a variety of basic movement and manipulative skills that are necessary to enjoy success in physical activity settings; develop the ability to get along with others in a movement environment; and enjoy and seek out physical activity. A complete list of the objectives for the healthy lifestyles, motor skills and movement knowledge, and social and personal skills development can be found on their web page at the click of the "About SPARK" link.

SPARK provides a wide range of services through their all-inclusive package, which is comprised of an assessment/evaluation; curricula, staff development, equipment, and follow-up/consultation. The SPARK curricula were written with consideration from curriculum experts, professional organizations and their standards, national and state guidelines, and Healthy Goals 2010. The lessons, which are marketed as practical and effective, come in three-ring binders that allow users to easily pull the lessons out and use them in practical locations. These come in six separate binders that can be purchased separately:

- *SPARK Early Childhood* (for children three- to five-years-old) – The youngsters work on their gross motor development, physical activity levels, social skills, and school readiness.
- *SPARK K-2 PE* (for kindergartners through second graders) – Fun warm-up activities get the students moving. Lessons within ten instructional units follow with themes like Dance with Me, Parachute Parade, and Bean Bag Boogie. Additionally, the curricula come with a literacy section and suggestions for integrating the academic areas.

- *SPARK 3-6 PE* (for the third through sixth grade youth) – Students build on what they learned from the K-2 curriculum. The instruction delivery is divided into two types of activities – health-related fitness and skill-related fitness – with a cool-down element. This curriculum includes personalized fitness tests, tips for academic integration, and social skills themes.
- *SPARK 6-8 PE* (for the middle school grades) – The unit is comprised of 20 chapters on a variety of traditional sports and physical activities like golf, Frisbee, and softball. However, these have been adapted so that there is greater student participation and enjoyment. Tips are also included for dealing with common PE obstacles such as lack of space or limited equipment, as well as tools to help teachers align their instruction with the state or professional standards.
- *SPARK Lifelong Wellness* (for two separate levels fourth and fifth graders and fifth and sixth graders) – This is the health promotion curricula where students learn nutrition and healthy food choices, goal setting, balance and moderation in diet and exercise, decreasing TV viewing, etc. There are 10 interactive, 20-minute lessons, with homework assignments that invite parents to participate with their children. The curriculum is organized into: Introduction and Overview, Lesson Plans, Copy Masters, Supplementary Lessons, and Outlines.
- *SPARK After School* (for Kindergarten through eighth grade) – There are over 450 pages of recreational activities ideal for youth leaders to use to involve students in Great Games, Dynamic Dances, Super Sports, and so forth. Practical tips for fitness activities, social skills building, making equipment, and more are included in the binder of activities.

Each of the curricula is about $90 and can be purchased through the SPARK website, which offers a wide-range of links that describe the program and curricula in much detail.

TAKE 10! Getting Kids Active
http://www.take10.net/

The "TAKE 10!" curriculum is intended for students in kindergarten through fifth grade and is meant to reduce the long periods of time that students spend sitting in their desks. "TAKE 10!" uses 10-minute physical activities to reinforce skills and concepts from the content areas (i.e., reading, math, social studies, and so forth) through movement. According to the website, the curriculum motivates students in non-traditional ways by addressing multiple learning styles thereby generating enthusiasm about being active outside the classroom. Additionally, a host of characters known as Organwise Guys (e.g., Hearty Heart, Sir Rebrum, Madame Muscle, Windy, and so forth) teach key concepts such as the importance of drinking water and the number of fruit and vegetables that should be eaten daily.

The materials kit for each specific grade level is available for $79 and includes:

- More than 30 multi-level activity cards that are closely linked to 50 worksheets;
- Posters and stickers to track student progress;
- Teacher resources; and
- Assessment and evaluation tools.

A slew of "TAKE 10!" incentives like pencils, stickers, t-shirts, messenger bags, and so forth can be purchased separately. The "TAKE 10!" product line includes teacher training resources, and a pre-k, middle school, and home curricula.

WHAT ARE SOME KEY ELEMENTS I SHOULD LOOK FOR WHEN EVALUATING A POTENTIAL PROGRAM?

When exploring different curricula to implement in your school or classroom use these essential elements as a guide to help you find the best program to fit your students' needs.

Essential Element #1. The Program Should Be Proven Effective

The program framework should encompass a well-defined curriculum that is standards-based with benchmarks that includes evaluation and assessment measures for all of the prescribed objectives. More importantly, the program should be known as an effective one proven through studies that are data-driven and statistically tested. Some programs may seem attractive, fun, appropriate, easy to administer, and possibly a wise choice, but could prove a waste of time or disastrous if there is no scientific basis for its effectiveness. In other words, ask yourself, "Have others had success with this program?" And, "How successful were they?" Failing to do so could lead to what seems as interminable and trivial instruction that has little or no positive effects on your students' health knowledge, skills, behavior, attitudes, and values.

Essential Element #2. The Program Framework Should Include A Family Component

The program should focus on all aspects of the student's life, not just at school. In order for teachers to help students develop positive long-lasting healthy habits, they need to enlist parental and familial support and understanding. After all, parents generally regulate what and how often their children eat and how they spend their free time. And, it is the family that sets the attitudes and behaviors toward eating and physical activity. Indeed, the family plays a key role in a youngster's health. To gain their support, the program should offer assignments and instructional activities that invite parents and family members to participate accordingly. By design, the program should encompass components that:

- Educate parents about the importance of nutrition and physical activity in everyday life;

- Reinforce concepts learned at school through homework and home-based projects;
- Encourage family members to support one another;
- Teach how to make their home environment a healthy one;
- Encourage parents to support their children in enjoyable physical activity;
- Promote the health and well-being message consistently across various environments; and
- Are culturally relevant.

Essential Element #3. The Program Framework Should Foster A Nurturing and Supportive Environment

The program should be fun, encouraging, motivating, inviting and does not single out youth, expect them to lose weight, force them to participate in activities they do not want to, or embarrass or humiliate them in any way. The goal in mind is to develop a healthy physical and mental body. Thus, the program framework should cultivate a positive self-esteem, a strong self-confidence, and a healthy body image. To enhance students' well-being, the program components should:

- Teach how to enhance, protect, and improve their self-esteem, self-confidence, and self-perception;
- Promote a positive body image and body satisfaction; and
- Teach about individual differences so that everyone is accepted and respected at any size.

Essential Element #4. The Program Framework Should Offer Ample Opportunities to Apply Health Knowledge, Skills, Attitudes, and Values

The program should incorporate instructional activities where students are actively learning about their health. In other words, students should practice making informed decisions that are consistent with a healthy lifestyle. Here is the opportunity for students to learn how the consequences of their behaviors now affect their current and future health status. As much as possible, they should be encouraged to apply healthy living concepts in their everyday lives. The program components should afford students the opportunities to practice life skills such as:

- Identifying the benefits of healthy habits;
- Making healthy selections;
- Promoting their own health and the health of those around;
- Maintaining their health;
- Identifying habits that work against good health;
- Setting realistic goals; and
- Tracking and monitoring progress.

Essential Element #5. The Program Framework Should Teach About and Promote Healthy Eating

The program should encompass hands-on lessons that teach about eating habits that are consistent with the *Dietary Guidelines for Americans* and *MyPyramid*. Students should learn about good nutrition, food variety, moderation, portion control, food labels, and so forth. The curriculum should be sequential, developmentally appropriate, and fun. To help students develop a positive attitude toward food, stress healthy food consumption through instruction that:

- Underscores the importance of a well-balanced diet;
- Teaches the recommended daily food allowance;
- Informs how to reduce fat, sugar, and sodium consumption and increase fiber intake;
- Teaches skills to resist nutrient inferior foods;
- Guides in assessing their current diet and their eating habits;
- Integrates the school food service; and
- Is personally relevant.

Essential Element #6. The Program Framework Should Promote Physical Activity Across Environments

The program should teach about the importance and benefits of physical activity and fitness and follow with ideas on how to become physically active at school, home, and in the community on a regular basis. The program should stress at least one hour of physical activity a day, which means that students have to learn that they have to fulfill this need at and away from school. The physical activity at school should actively engage the students at least half of the time, and be fun, enjoyable, and inviting. This can be accomplished by offering a range of creative and traditional games, sports, exercise, and recreational activities during recess, physical education (where they can also learn about through fundamental motor skills development, sports, and so forth), after-school programs, school-based team sports, and community-based recreation. These activities should vary between a cooperative, competitive, and individualistic nature and allow them to experience some success so that they become encouraged to pursue their physical activity preference. So that students incorporate physical activity in their everyday life, seek a program that will be meaningful to your students with components that:

- Increase awareness that physical activity is beneficial;
- Help them explore leisure and recreational activities;
- Encourage safe physical activity that is appropriately challenging;
- Teach the importance of setting goals, practicing, and working out;
- Teach how to overcome common barriers of engaging in physical activity and how to fit it in their lives;
- Encourage students to participate fully in moderate to vigorous activities;

- Teach them to reflect on their own physical fitness and how to improve their performance;
- Build their confidence in physical activity;
- Reduce their screen time;
- Incorporate team-building exercises where they develop interpersonal skills;
- Empowers them to map out times when they can engage in physical activity;
- Complements academic instruction with physical activity;
- Is consistent with the national standards for physical education; and
- Is developmentally appropriate.

Essential Element #7. The Program Framework Should Address the Influence of External Factors on Eating and Physical Activity

Look for programs that explore the effect media and advertising have on students' choices. Students should learn about the purposes of commercials and ads and how they influence society to make fast, junk, and nutrient inferior food purchases. The program components should teach students the skills to resist social pressures including celebrity-endorsed messages and peer pressures with their own normative messages like, "This is the latest diet," or "Everybody's smoking to stay thin." The instruction should provide them an education on:

- The effects television can have on their eating habits and physical activity level;
- The effects media can have on self-esteem;
- Validating the claims made by some products and fad diets;
- The harmful effects of risky behaviors like smoking and alcohol use;
- Risky social situations and the implications of making bad decisions; and
- How to counter risky behaviors and situations with decision-making skills that lead to positive results.

CONCLUSION

Given the surge in childhood obesity, it seems that children are eating more and exercising less. These unhealthy decisions are not deliberate; many youth simply lack the knowledge to make the right choices, which is why it is so important to teach them basic health concepts. Key to improving their well-being is to empower them with the skills to eat right and exercise more. Many educational tools are available to help them balance diet and physical activity in their daily lives. Instructional resources for school and home often offer exciting ideas replete with interactive websites, lesson plans, posters, handouts, worksheets, and so forth. While some of the curricula can be purchased for a nominal fee, others are free. Whichever curriculum is chosen to meet your students' unique needs, it should be a proven effective program. Additionally, it should be developmentally appropriate, meaningful and nurturing, and promote good habits that youth can weave into their daily life. In all, these programs hold the potential to positively change their lives forever.

NOTES

[i] Source: East Carolina University Activity Promotion Laboratory. (2007). *Energizers: Classroom-based Physical Activities.* Retrieved June 25, 2007, from http://www.ncpe4me.com/pdf_files/K-5-Energizers.pdf. Reprinted with permission.

[ii] Source: Adapted from KidsHealth. (2007). *Nutrition & Fitness.* Retrieved June 25, 2007, from http://kidshealth.org/parent/nutrition_fit/index.html.

RESOURCES

At the risk of sounding redundant, childhood obesity is an epidemic. As many as 30% of children between 6- and 19-years-old are considered overweight. Make no mistake about it; these are real youth who could develop real health problems—including socio-emotional ones—if nothing is done to help them. Youth advocates, school personnel, and parents must collaborate to reduce obesity because children and youth cannot do it on their own. This can be accomplished by mobilizing informational resources that can lead to developing well-balanced programs inclusive of diet management, physical activity, and behavior modification. This chapter presents some resources that expand on childhood obesity and/or inform how to promote health and wellness. Particularly, the chapter answers:

- What are some print resources devoted to childhood obesity and health?
- What are some online resources on childhood obesity and health?
- What are some advocacy organizations, associations, and government agencies devoted to childhood obesity and health?

WHAT ARE SOME PRINT RESOURCES DEVOTED TO CHILHOOD OBESITY AND HEALTH?

Print resources abound to deepen the understanding of the current health status of youth. In fact, many offer the most recent information on developmentally appropriate teaching practices leading toward health and wellness. Consult some of the books and journal articles listed below to empower youth to commit their lifetime to making healthy and responsible decisions.

Books

The following books discourse childhood obesity. Notice by their titles that some are more general in nature; others deal specifically with trying to help youth develop positive lifelong habits.

Childhood obesity and health research
Richard K. Flamenbaum (2006)
Nova Science Publishers

Dr. Spear's lean kids: Lifestyle, exercise, attitude, nutrition
William Spears, Peter Spears, and Sean Foy (2003)
New American Library

Fed Up! Winning the war against childhood obesity
Susan Okie (2006)
National Academy Press

Generation extra large: Rescuing our children from the epidemic of obesity
Lisa Tartamella (2004)
Basic Books

Our overweight children: What parents, schools, and communities can do to control the fatness epidemic
Sharon Dalton (2004)
University of California Press

Overcoming childhood obesity
Colleen A. Thompson, & Ellen L. Shanley (2004)
Bull Publishing Company

Overcoming obesity in childhood and adolescence: A guide for school leaders
Donald Schumacher, & J. Allen Queen (2006)
Corwin Press

Overweight child: Promoting fitness and self-esteem
Teresa Pitman, & Miriam Kaufman (2000)
Firefly

A parent's guide to childhood obesity: A road map to health
American Academy of Pediatrics, & Sandra G. Hassink (2006)
American Academy of Pediatrics

Preventing childhood obesity: Health in the balance
Institute of Medicine Committee on Prevention of Obesity in Children and Youth, Catharyn T. Liverman, Vivica I. Kraak, & Jeffrey P. Koplan (2005)
National Academy Press

Progress in preventing childhood obesity: How do we measure up?
Jeffrey P. Koplan, Catharyn T. Liverman, Vivica I. Kraak, & Shannon L. Wisham (2007)
National Academies Press

Rescuing the emotional lives of overweight children: What our kids go through - and how we can help
Sylvia Rimm, & Eric Rimm (2005)
Rodale Books

Save your child from the fat epidemic: 7 steps every parent can take to ensure healthy, fit children for life
Gayle Povis Alleman, (1999)
Prima Publishing

Underage & overweight: America's childhood obesity crises – what every family needs to know
Francis M. Berg (2004)
Hatherleigh Press

Understanding childhood obesity
J. Clinton Smith (1999)
University Press of Mississippi

Your child's weight: Helping without harming
Ellyn Satter (2005)
Kelcy Press

Selected Journal Articles

The journal articles listed below are ideal for readers who seek to learn more about childhood obesity. Some of these are research-based articles that employ scientific methodology, while others are more discussant pieces that offer practical suggestions and information. In all, these may be worthwhile to circulate at conferences or training sessions to inform others about the crisis.

Agras, W., Hammer, L., McNicholas, F., & Kraemer, H. (2004). Risk factors for childhood overweight: A prospective study from birth to 9.5 years. *Journal of Pediatrics, 145(1),* 20-25.

American Academy of Pediatrics. (2001). Committee on public education: Children, adolescents, and television. *Pediatrics, 107(2),* 423-426.

American Academy of Pediatrics. (2003). Prevention of pediatric overweight and obesity. *Pediatrics, 112(2),* 424-430

American Academy of Pediatrics. (2003). Policy statement: Prevention of pediatric overweight and obesity. *Pediatrics, 112(2),* 424-430.

American Academy of Pediatrics. (2006). Children, Adolescents and Advertising. *Pediatrics, 118(6),* 2563-2569.

Anderson, R., Crespo, C., Bartlett, S., Cheskin, L., & Pratt. (1998). Relationship of physical activity and television watching with body weight and level of fatness among children: Results from the Third National Health and Nutrition Examination Survey. *JAMA, 279(12),* 938-942.

Baranowski, T., Cullen, K., Nicklas, T., Thompson, D., & Baranowski, J. (2002). School-based obesity prevention: A blueprint for taming the epidemic. *American Journal of Health Behaviors, 26(6),* 486-493.

Barlow, S., & Dietz, W. (1998). Obesity evaluation and treatment: Expert committee recommendations. *Pediatrics, 102(3),* 1-11.

Biddle, S., Gorely, T., & Stensel, D. (2004). Health enhancing physical activity and sedentary behaviour in children and adolescents. *Journal of Sports Sciences, 22(8),* 679-703.

Broadwater, H. (2002). Reshaping the future for overweight kids. *RN, 65(11),* 36-41.

Burgeson, C., Wechsler, H., Brener, N., Young, J., & Spain, C. (2003). Physical education and activity: Results from the school health policies and programs study 2000. *The Journal of Physical Education, 24(2),* 111-118.

Coles, A. (2004, May/June). Generation XXL. Obesity among U.S. schoolchildren is on the rise, and schools can fight this battle of the bulge. *American Teacher,* pp. 6-7.

Council on Sports Medicine and Fitness and Council on School Health. (2006). Active healthy living: prevention of childhood obesity through increased physical activity. *Pediatrics, 117(5),* 1834-1842.

Covington, C., Cybulski, M., Davis, T., Duca, G., Farrell, E., Kasgorgis, M., Kator, C., & Sell, T. (2001). Kids on the move: Preventing obesity among urban children. *American Journal of Nursing, 101(3),* 73-81.

Crespo, C., & Arbesman, J. (2003). Obesity in the United States: A worrisome epidemic. *Physician & Sportsmedicine, 31(11),* 23-28.

Datar, A., & Sturm, R. (2004). Physical education in elementary school and body mass index: Evidence from the early childhood longitudinal study. *American Journal of Public Health, 94(9),* 1501-1505.

Davis, S., Davis, M., Northington, L., Moll, G., & Kolar, K. (2002). Childhood obesity reduction by school based programs. *The ABNF Journal,* 145-149.

Deckelbaum, R., & Williams, C. (2001). Childhood obesity: The health issue. *Obesity Research, 9(4)*, 239-243.

Dennison, B., Erb, T., & Jenkins, P. (2002). Television viewing and television in bedroom associated with overweight risk among low-income preschool children. *Pediatrics, 109(6)*, e16.

Dietz, W. (1998). Health consequences of obesity in youth: Childhood predictors of adult diseases. *Pediatrics, 75(5)*, 807-812.

Drohan, S. (2002). Managing early childhood obesity in the primary care setting: A behavior modification approach. *Pediatric Nursing, 28(6)*, 599-610.

Evans, W., Finkelstein, E., Kamerow, D., & Renaud, J. (2005). Public perceptions of childhood obesity. *American Journal of Preventive Medicine, 28(1)*, 26-32.

Feeg, V. (2004). Combating childhood obesity: A collective effort. *Pediatric Nursing, 30(5)*, 361-362.

Flodmark, C., Marcus, C., & Britton, M. (2006). Interventions to prevent obesity in children and adolescents: a systematic literature review. *International Journal of Obesity, 30(4)*, 579-589.

Fowler-Brown, A., & Kahwati, L. (2004). Prevention and treatment of overweight in children and adolescents. *American Family Physician, 69(11)*, 2591-2598.

Freedman, D., Khan, L., Serdula, M., Ogden, C., & Dietz, W. (2006). Racial and ethnic differences in secular trends for childhood BMI, weight, and height. *Obesity, 14(2)*, 301-308.

Fren, M., Malin, S., Bansal, N., Delgado, M., Greer, Y., Havice, M., Ho, M., & Schweizer, H. (2003). Addressing health disparities in middle school students' nutrition and exercise. *Journal of Community Health Nursing, 20(1)*, 1-14.

Fuhr, J., & Barclay, K. (1999). The importance of appropriate nutrition and nutrition education. *Young Children, 53(1)*, 74-80.

Gable, S., & Lutz, S. (2000). Household, parent, and child contributions to childhood obesity. *Family Relations, 49(3)*, 293-300.

Gillis, L., Kennedy, L., Gillis, A., & Bar-Or, O. (2002). Relationship between juvenile obesity, dietary energy and fat intake and physical activity. *International Journal of Obesity, 26(4)*, 458-463.

Goodman, E., Hinden, B., & Khandlewal, S. (2000). Accuracy of teen and parental reports of obesity and body mass index. *Pediatrics, 106 (1)*, 52-58.

Grunbaum, J., Kann, L., Kinchen, S., Ross, J., Hawkins, J., Lowry, R., Harris, W., McManus, T., Chyen, D., & Collins, J. (2004). Youth risk behavior surveillance – United States, 2003. *Morbidity and Mortality Weekly Report, 53(2),* 1-95.

Inge, T., et al. (2004). Bariatric Surgery for Severely Overweight Adolescents: Concerns and Recommendations. *Pediatrics, 114(1),* 217-23.

Jonides, L., Buschbacher, V., & Barlow, S. (2002). Management of child and adolescent obesity: Psychological, emotional, and behavioral assessment. *Pediatrics, 110(1),* 215-221.

Lederman, S., Akabas, S., & Moore, B. (2004). Editor's overview of the conference on preventing childhood obesity. *Pediatrics, 114(4),* 1139-1145.

Louie, D., Sanchez, E., Faircloth, S., & Dietz, W. (2003). School-based policies: Nutrition and physical activity. *Journal of Law, Medicine, and Ethics, 31(4) (special supplement),* 73-75.

Lowry, R., Wechsler, H., Galuska, D., Fulton, J., & Kann, L. (2002). Television viewing and its association with overweight, sedentary lifestyle, and insufficient consumption of fruits and vegetables among US high school students: Difference by race, ethnicity, and gender. *Journal of School Health, 72(10),* 413-421.

Lumeng, J., Rahnama, S., Appugliese, D., Kaciroti, N., & Bradley, R. (2006). Television exposure and overweight risk in preschoolers. *Archives of Pediatric and Adolescent Medicine, 160(4),* 417-422.

Lynn-Garbe, C., & Hoot, J. (2005). Weighing in on the issue of childhood obesity. *Childhood Education, 81(2),* 70-76.

Maddock, J. (2004). The relationship between obesity and the prevalence of fast food restaurants: State-level analysis. *American Journal of Health Promotion, 19(2),* 137-143.

Marr, L. (2004). Soft drinks, childhood overweight, and the role of nutrition educators: Let's base our solutions on reality and sound science. *Journal of Nutrition Education and Behavior, 36(5),* 258-263.

Matheson, D., Killen, J., Wang, Y., Varady, A., & Robinson, T. (2004). Children's food consumption during television viewing. *American Journal of Clinical Nutrition, 79(6),* 1088-1094.

McMurray, R., Harrell, J., Bangdiwala, S., Bradley, C., Deng, S., & Levine, A. (2002). A school-based intervention can reduce body fat and blood pressure in young adolescents. *Journal of Adolescent Medicine, 31(2),* 125-132.

Ogden, C., Carroll, M., Curtin, L., McDowell, M., Tabak, C., & Flegal, K. (2006). Prevalence of overweight and obesity in the United States, 1999-2004. *JAMA, 295(13),* 1549-1555.

Olshansky, S., et al. (2005). A potential decline in life expectancy in the United States in the 21st century. *New England Journal of Medicine, 252(11),* 1138-1145.

Pate, R., Pfeiffer, K., Trost, S., Ziegler, P., & Dowda, M. (2004). Physical activity among children attending preschools. *Pediatrics, 114(5),* 1258-1263.

Ribeiro, J., Guerra, S., Pinto, A., Oliveira, J., Duarte, J., & Mota, J. (2003). Overweight and obesity in children and adolescents: Relationships with blood pressure, and physical activity. *Annals of Human Biology, 30(2),* 203-213.

Salsberry, P., & Reagan P. (2005). Dynamics of Early Childhood Overweight. *Pediatrics, 116(6),* 1329-1338.

Speiser, P., et al. (2005). Consensus Statement: Childhood Obesity. *Journal of Clinical Endocrinolgy & Metabolism, 90(3),* 1871-1887.

Strauss, R. (2000). Childhood obesity and self-esteem. *Pediatrics, 105(4),* e15.

Strock, G., Cottrell, E., Abang, A., Buschbacher, R., & Hannon, T. (2005). Childhood obesity: A simple equation with complex variables. *Journal of Long-term Effects of Medical Implants, 15(1),* 15-32.

Taylor, K. (2003). Food fights: Schools, students, and the law. *Principal Leadership, 3(6),* 63-66.

Troicano, R., & Flegal, K. (1998). Overweight children and adolescents: Description, epidemiology, and demographics. *Pediatrics, 101(3),* 497-504.

Vail, K. (2004). Obesity epidemic. *American School Board Journal, 191(1),* 22-25.

Weiss, R., Dziura, J., Burgert, T., Tamborlane, W., Taksali, S., Yeckel, C., Allen, K., Lopes, M., Savoye, M., Morrison, J., Sherwin, R., & Caprio, S. (2004). Obesity and the metabolic syndrome in children and adolescents. *New England Journal of Medicine, 350(23),* 2362-2374.

Welsh, J., Cogswell, M., Rogers, S., Mei, Z., & Grummer-Strawn, L. (2005). Overweight among low-income preschool children associated with the consumption of sweet drinks: Missouri, 1999-2002. *Pediatrics, 115(2),* 223-e229.

Wu, F., Yu, S., Wei, I, & Yin, T. (2003). Weight-control behavior among obese children: association with family-related factors. *Journal of Nursing Research, 11(1),* 19-28.

Zwiauer, K. (2000). Prevention and treatment of overweight and obesity in children and adolescents. *Europe Journal of Pediatrics, 59(S1),* 56-68.

WHAT ARE SOME ONLINE RESOURCES ON CHILHOOD OBESITY AND HEALTH?

The Internet offers a sea of resources on childhood obesity and the closely tied topic of health and well-being, which can be used to positively influence students to protect their own health. Some of these resources can be found below under the following divisions: Websites; Interactive Resources; Tips and Guidelines; Electronically Accessible Reports; and fact sheets.

Wesites

There are a number of websites that offer valuable resources to guide consumers toward healthier lives. The sites listed below furnish site visitors with information on the varying dimensions of health, which can then be used to increase students' health knowledge, behavior, and attitudes.

Action For Healthy Kids
www.actionforhealthykids.org

Active Living By Design
www.activelivingbydesign.org

America Bikes
www.americabikes.org

America on the Move
aom.americaonthemove.org

America Walks
www.americawalks.com

Centers for Disease Control and Prevention, Division of Nutrition and Physical Activity
www.cdc.gov/nccdphp/dnpa/index.htm

Child and Adolescent Nutrition Knowledge Path
www.mchlibrary.info/KnowledgePaths/kp_childnutr.html

Face the Fats!
www.americanheart.org/presenter.jhtml?identifier=3046074

Girls on the Run
www.girlsontherun.org

Hallmark Healthy High 5
www.highmarkhealthyhigh5.org

Healthy People 2010
www.healthypeople.gov/Publications

Healthy Weight Network
www.healthyweight.net

Hearts N/ Parks (National Heart, Lung, and Blood Institute)
www.nhlbi.nih.gov/health/prof/heart/obesity/hrt_n_pk/index.htm

Kidshape
www.kidshape.com

KidSource Online - Promoting Physical Activity and Exercise among Children
www.kidsource.com/kidsource/content4/promote.phyed.html

Maternal and Child Health Library
www.mchlibrary.info

MyPyramid.gov
www.mypyramid.gov

No Junk Food
www.nojunkfood.org

Obesity Education Initiative
www.nhlbi.nih.gov/about/oei/index.htm

Obesity Law and Advocacy Center
www.obesitylaw.com

PE Central
www.pecentral.org

Pelink4u – Promoting Active and Healthy Lifestyles
www.pelinks4u.org

Project Fit America
www.projectfitamerica.org

Powerful Girls Have Powerful Bones
www.cdc.gov/powerfulbones/index.html

Safe Routes to School
www.bikewalk.org

Shaping America's Youth
www.shapingamericasyouth.com

Steps to a Healthier US
www.healthierus.gov

USDA, Food & Nutrition Information Center
www.nal.usda.gov/fnic/dga/rda.htm

USDA, Healthy Meals Resource System
healthymeals.nal.usda.gov

USDA, Team Nutrition
www.fns.usda.gov/tn

The United Health Foundation
www.unitedhealthfoundation.org/mouth.html

Vegeterianteen
www.vegetariantcen.com

Youth Fitness Curriculum
www.acefitness.org/ofk/youthFitness

Interactive Resources

Following is a list of websites that are designed to interface with site visitors. Some of these are more serious, like the BMI calculators that will compute the BMI of adults and youth or the databases that will retrieve past and current information on state and federal legislation. The others are fun-natured and meant to educate site visitors with amusing quizzes on significant pieces of information.

BMI Percentile Calculator for Child and Teen
http://apps.nccd.cdc.gov/dnpabmi/Calculator.aspx

CDC BMI Calculators
http://apps.nccd.cdc.gov/dnpabmi/Calculator.aspx

Calculate Your Body Mass Index
www.nhlbisupport.com/bmi

Database of state nutrition and physical activity legislation
http://apps.nccd.cdc.gov/DNPALeg/

Database of state physical activity and nutrition legislation
http://www.ncsl.org/programs/health/pp/healthpromo.cfm

Feed the Face
http://www.cspinet.org/cgi-bin/smartmouth/feedtheface.pl

How do your favorite food snack stack up?
http://www.cspinet.org/cgi-bin/smartmouth/choose.pl

Junk Food Quiz
http://www.cspinet.org/nutritionpolicy/junkfoodquiz.html

Portion Distortion Quiz
http://hin.nhlbi.nih.gov/portion/index.htm

Quiz Yourself! Test Your Food Label Knowledge!
http://www.cfsan.fda.gov/~dms/flquiz1.html

Restaurant Quiz
http://www.cspinet.org/nutritionpolicy/restaurant_quiz.html

USDA, National Nutrient Database for Standard Reference
http://www.nal.usda.gov/fnic/foodcomp/search/

Tips and Guidelines

Listed below are some "how-to" leaflet-like materials that are ideal for building healthy communities, whether at home, school, or in the classroom. Consult these for practical ideas on how to get and stay healthy or build environments that enhance the health of children and adolescents.

Alternatives to Using Food As a Reward
http://www.tn.fcs.msue.msu.edu/foodrewards.pdf

Classroom Party Ideas
http://www.cspinet.org/nutritionpolicy/classroompartyideasCA.pdf

169

Constructive Classroom Rewards: Promoting Good Habits While Protecting Children's Health
http://www.cspinet.org/nutritionpolicy/constructive_rewards.pdf

Food Free Celebrations
http://www.cspinet.org/nutritionpolicy/mphaideas.pdf

Guidelines for Collecting Heights and Weights on Children and Adolescents in School Settings
www.CNR.Berkeley.EDU/cwh/resources/childrenandweight.shtml

Guidelines for School and Community Programs to Promote Lifelong Physical Activity Among Young People
ftp://ftp.cdc.gov/pub/Publications/mmwr/rr/rr4606.pdf

Guidelines for School Health Programs to Promote Lifelong Healthy Eating
ftp://ftp.cdc.gov/pub/Publications/mmwr/rr/rr4509.pdf

Healthy Celebrations
http://www.cspinet.org/nutritionpolicy/healthycelebrationsCT.pdf

Healthy Eating and Physical Activity Across Your Lifespan: Helping Your Child
www.niddk.nih.gov/health/nutrit/pubs/parentips/tipsforparents.htm

Healthy School Snacks
http://www.cspinet.org/nutritionpolicy/healthy_school_snacks.pdf

KidsWalk-to-School: A Guide to Promote Walking to School
http://www.cdc.gov/nccdphp/dnpa/kidswalk/pdf/kidswalk.pdf

Model School Wellness Policies
http://www.schoolwellnesspolicies.org/

School Foods Toolkit
www.cspinet.org/schoolfood/index.html

Shape of the Nation
http://www.aahperd.org/NASPE/ShapeOfTheNation/PDF/ShapeOfTheNation.pdf

Start Healthy: the Guide to Teaching Your Little One Good Eating Habits
http://www.eatright.org/ada/files/gerber.pdf

Tips for Using the Food Guide Pyramid for Young Children 2 to 6 Years Old
www.usda.gov/cnpp/KidsPyra/PyrBook.pdf

What's a Mom to Do? Healthy Eating Tips for Families
http://www.eatright.org/ada/files/Wendys.pdf

Electronically Accessible Reports

Below are some reports and studies that can be accessed on the web. While many of them are commissioned investigations that enlighten readers about varying aspects of the obesity issue, others are reports on how to maintain a healthy lifestyle complete with ideas on how to improve diet and increase physical activity.

35 Years: Building a Healthier America Since 1971
http://www.cspinet.org/CSPI_35thAR.pdf

Action Plan: Healthy People 2010 Objectives for Prevention and Control of Childhood Obesity
www.apha.org/ppp/obesity_toolkit/005_action_plan.htm

Active Healthy Living: Prevention of Childhood Obesity Through Increased Physical Activity
http://www.aap.org/obesity/recommendations.htm

A Healthier You
http://www.health.gov/dietaryguidelines/dga2005/healthieryou/contents.htm

Anyone's Guess: The Need for Nutrition Labeling at Fast-Food and Other Chain Restaurants
http://www.cspinet.org/restaurantreport.pdf

Barriers to Children Walking to or from School --- United States, 2004
http://www.cdc.gov/mmwr/preview/mmwrhtml/mm5438a2.htm

Calories Count: Report of the Working Group on Obesity
http://www.cfsan.fda.gov/~dms/owg-toc.html

Childhood Obesity: A Lifelong Threat to Health
http://www.georgetown.edu/research/ihcrp/agingsociety/pdfs/obesity.pdf

Childhood Obesity: Factors Affecting Physical Activity
http://www.gao.gov/new.items/d07260r.pdf

Dispensing Junk: How School Vending Undermines Efforts to Feed Children Well
http://www.cspinet.org/new/pdf/dispensing_junk.pdf

Sweet Deals: School Fundraising Can be Healthy and Profitable
http://www.cspinet.org/new/pdf/schoolfundraising.pdf

Dietary Guidelines for Americans, 2005
http://www.health.gov/dietaryguidelines/dga2005/document/default.htm

Engaging School Leaders as Partners in Creating Healthy Schools
http://www.actionforhealthykids.org/pdf/AFHK%20Leaders%20Guide%20FINAL
3_5.pdf

*F as in Fat: How Obesity Policies are Failing in America. Trust for America's
Health*
http://healthyamericans.org/reports/obesity/ObesityExecSum.pdf

*Finding Your Way to a Healthier You: Based on the Dietary Guidelines for
Americans*
http://www.health.gov/dietaryguidelines/dga2005/document/html/brochure.htm

*Food Sold in competition with USDA school meal programs: A report to Congress
USDA*
http://www.fns.usda.gov/cnd/Lunch/CompetitiveFoods/report_congress.htm

*Foundation for the Future II: Analysis Local Wellness Policies from 140 School
Districts in 49 States*
http://www.schoolnutrition.org/uploadedFiles/SchoolNutrition.org/News_&_Publi
cations/School_Foodservice_News/New_Folder/Regional%20LWP%20Report.pdf

*From the Top Down: Engaging School Leaders in Creating a Healthier, More
Physically Active School Environment*
http://www.actionforhealthykids.org/pdf/SchoolLeaders_FR_1219Final.pdf

From Wallet to Waistline: The Hidden Cost of Super Sizing
http://www.cspinet.org/w2w.pdf

*Giving Kids the Voice of Authority: Engaging Students in the Fight Against
Childhood   Obesity*
http://www.actionforhealthykids.org/pdf/Students_FR_91FINAL.pdf

Health, United States, 2006 with Chartbook on Trends in the Health of Americans
http://www.cdc.gov/nchs/data/hus/hus06.pdf

Healthy Schools for Healthy Kids
http://www.rwjf.org/files/publications/other/HealthySchools.pdf

Ideas, Commitment, Action, Results: Model Projects Advancing the Cause of School Wellness

http://www.actionforhealthykids.org/pdf/AFHK%20Field%20Report%20Vol%202%20No%201%20FINAL%20PDF.pdf

The Importance of Playing in Promoting Healthy Child Development and Maintaining Strong Parent-Child Bonds
http://www.acefitness.org/ofk/youthFitness/

The Learning Connection: The Value of Improving Nutrition and Physical Activity in Our Schools

http://www.actionforhealthykids.org/pdf/Learning%20Connection%20-%20Full%20Report%20001006.pdf

The Media Family: Electronic Media in the Lives of Infants, Toddlers, Preschoolers and Their Parents
http://www.kff.org/entmedia/upload/7500.pdf

Pediatric Nutrition Surveillance
http://www.cdc.gov/pednss/pdfs/PedNSS_2003_Summary.pdf

Pestering Parents: How Food Companies Market Obesity to Children
http://www.cspinet.org/new/pdf/pesteringparentsnopictures.pdf

Physical Activity Evaluation Handbook
http://www.cdc.gov/nccdphp/dnpa/physical/health_professionals/interventions/handbook.pdf

Promoting Better Health for Young People through Physical Activity and Sports: A Report to the President
http://www.cdc.gov/healthyyouth/physicalactivity/promoting_health/

Public Attitudes toward Physical Education
http://www.aahperd.org/naspe/pdf_files/whatsnew-survey.pdf

Public Health Strategies for Preventing and Controlling Overweight and Obesity in School and Worksite Settings: A Report on Recommendations of the Task Force on Community Preventive Services
http://www.cdc.gov/mmwr/preview/mmwrhtml/rr5410a1.htm

Quarterly Report on State Legislation and Policies Affecting Child and Adolescent Nutrition, Obesity and Physical Activity
http://www.rwjf.org/files/research/NCSL%20FinalApril%202006%20Report.pdf

Overweight Children and Youth
http://www.childtrendsdatabank.org/pdf/15_PDF.pdf

Reducing Children's TV Time to Reduce the Risk of Childhood Overweight: The Children's Media Use Study
http://www.cdc.gov/nccdphp/dnpa/obesity/pdf/TV_Time_Highligts.pdf

The Role of Media in Childhood Obesity
http://www.kff.org/entmedia/upload/The-Role-Of-Media-in-Childhood-Obesity.pdf

Salt Assault: Brand-name Comparisons of Processed Foods
http://www.cspinet.org/new/pdf/salt_report_update.pdf

Secondary School Health Education Related to Nutrition and Physical Activity --- Selected Sites, United States, 2004
http://www.cdc.gov/mmwr/preview/mmwrhtml/mm5530a2.htm

Socioeconomic Determinants of Healthy Eating Habits and Physical Activity Levels Among Adolescents
http://www.shapingamericasyouth.com/WHOHBSCForum2006_ProceedingsRepo rt_v14June06.pdf?cid=283

Strategic Plan for Obesity Research
http://obesityresearch.nih.gov/About/Obesity_EntireDocument.pdf

The Surgeon General's Call to Action to Prevent and Decrease Overweight and Obesity 2000
http://www.surgcongeneral.gov/topics/obesity/

Tapping Into the Power: Engaging Parents in the Fight Against Childhood Obesity
http://www.actionforhealthykids.org/pdf/Parents%20FR_823FINAL.pdf

Toolkit for Health Professionals
http://www.health.gov/dietaryguidelines/dga2005/toolkit/default.htm

Weighing In: Helping Girls be Healthy Today, Healthy Tomorrow
http://www.girlscouts.org/research/pdf/weighing_in.pdf

Fact Sheets

Assorted fact sheets follow that provide statistics on childhood obesity, public health, as well as background information to engender habits that lead to long-term healthy habits. These are excellent tools to use to publicize the message that childhood obesity is a crisis that needs pre-eminent attention.

Advertising, Marketing, and the Media: Improving Messages
http://www.iom.edu/Object.File/Master/22/609/fact%20sheet%20-%20marketing%20finaBitticks.pdf

Benefits of Having a Recess Before Lunch Policy and Tips for Getting Started
http://www.cspinet.org/nutritionpolicy/recessbrochure.pdf

Benefits of School Meal Participation
http://www.actionforhealthykids.org/filelib/facts_and_findings/Benefits%20of%20School%20Meal%20Participation.pdf

Better Nutrition and Physical Activity Can Boost Achievement and School's Bottom Line
http://www.actionforhealthykids.org/pdf/Learning%20Connection%20FS.pdf

Building the Argument: Providing Health-Promoting Foods Throughout Our Schools
http://www.actionforhealthykids.org/filelib/facts_and_findings/Providing%20Health%20Promoting%20Foods.pdf

Building the Argument: The Need for Physical Education and Physical Activity in Our Schools
http://www.actionforhealthykids.org/filelib/facts_and_findings/Need%20for%20PE-PA.pdf

Childhood Obesity in the United States: Facts and Figures
http://www.iom.edu/Object.File/Master/22/606/FINALfactsandfigures2.pdf

Childhood Obesity the Preventable Threat to America's Youth
http://www.actionforhealthykids.org/filelib/facts_and_findings/Childhood%20Obesity%20Fact%20Sheet%20Revised%207-29-05.pdf

Fast Facts on U.S. Public Schools
http://www.actionforhealthykids.org/filelib/facts_and_findings/Fast%20Stats%20on%20U.%20S.%20Public%20Schools.pdf

Health Effects of Obesity
http://obesity1.tempdomainname.com/subs/fastfacts/Health_Effects.shtml

Obesity in the U.S.
http://obesity1.tempdomainname.com/subs/fastfacts/obesity_US.shtml

Obesity in Youth
http://obesity1.tempdomainname.com/subs/fastfacts/obesity_youth.shtml

Overview of the IOM's Childhood Obesity Study
http://www.iom.edu/Object.File/Master/22/604/fact%20sheet%20-%20overview%20finalBitticks.pdf

Parents Can Play a Role in Preventing Childhood Obesity
http://www.iom.edu/Object.File/Master/22/617/Fact%20Sheet%20-%20Home%20FINALBitticks.pdf

The Role of Sound Nutrition and Physical Activity in Academic Achievement
http://www.actionforhealthykids.org/filelib/facts_and_findings/nutrition,%20physical%20activity%20and%20achievement.pdf

Schools Can Play a Role in Preventing Childhood Obesity
http://www.iom.edu/Object.File/Master/22/615/Fact%20Sheet%20-%20Schools%20FINALBitticks.pdf

State School Nutrition Legislation Supports Parental and Local Control
http://www.cspinet.org/nutritionpolicy/statelocal_controlfactsheet.pdf

Update USDA's School Nutrition Standards for Foods and Beverages Sold Outside of School Meals
http://www.cspinet.org/nutritionpolicy/fedschoolfoods.pdf

Wellness Policy Fact Sheet
http://www.actionforhealthykids.org/filelib/facts_and_findings/Wellness%20Fact%20Sheet%209-21-05.pdf

Wellness Policy Fact Sheet
http://www.aap.org/obesity/WellnessPolicyFactSheet.pdf

What is obesity?
http://obesity1.tempdomainname.com/subs/fastfacts/obesity_what2.shtml

WHAT ARE SOME ADVOCACY ORGANIZATIONS, ASSOCIATIONS, AND GOVERNMENT AGENCIES DEVOTED TO CHILDHOOD OBESITY AND HEALTH?

Listed below are some organizations, associations, and government agencies that strive to educate the public about the childhood obesity crises. The cardinal goal for this coalition is to improve the health of citizens nationwide by offering sorts of campaign materials ranging from nutrition to exercise. Many of the respective websites provide resources that are specific to their cause (e.g., cardiovascular disease prevention), while the information that others afford is more general with ideas on how to inhibit childhood obesity. Explore these websites for additional fact sheets, reports and studies, guidelines, and so forth.

American Academy of Kinesiology and Physical Education
P.O. Box 5076
Champaign, IL 61820
(800) 747-4457
www.aakpe.org

American Academy of Pediatrics
141 Northwest Point Blvd.
Elk Grove Village, IL 60007
(847) 434-4000
www.aap.org

American Alliance for Health, Physical Education, Recreation, and Dance
1900 Association Drive
Reston, Virginia 20191
(800) 213-7193
www.aahperd.org

American Association of Family and Consumer Sciences
400 N. Columbus Street, Suite 202
Alexandria, VA 22314
(703) 706.4600
www.aafcs.org

American College of Sports Medicine
401 West Michigan Street
Indianapolis, IN 46202
(317) 637-9200
www.acsm.org

American Council for Fitness and Nutrition
P.O. Box 33396
Washington, DC 20033
(800) 953-1700
www.acfn.org

American Council on Exercise
4851 Paramount Drive
San Diego, California 92123
(858) 279-8227
www.acefitness.org

American Diabetes Association
1701 North Beauregard Street
Alexandria, VA 22311
(800) 342-2383
www.diabetes.org

American Dietetic Association
120 South Riverside Plaza, Suite 2000
Chicago, Illinois 60606
(800) 877-1600
www.eatright.org

American Heart Association
7272 Greenville Avenue
Dallas, TX 75231
(800) 242-8721
www.americanheart.org

American Medical Association
515 N. State Street
Chicago, IL 60610
(800) 621-8335
www.ama-assn.org

American Public Health Association
800 I Street, NW
Washington, DC 20001
(202) 777-2742
www.apha.org

American School Food Service Association
700 South Washington Street, Suite 300
Alexandria, VA 22314
(703) 739-3900
www.asfsa.org

American School Health Association
7263 State Route 43
P.O. Box 708
Kent, Ohio 44240
(330) 678-1601
www.ashaweb.org

Association for Community Health Improvement
180 Montgomery Street, Suite 1520
San Francisco, CA 94104
(415) 248.8408
www.communityhlth.org

Center for Health and Health Care in Schools
2121 K Street, NW Suite 250
Washington, DC 20036
(202) 466-3396
www.healthinschools.org/publications.asp

Center for Science in the Public Interest
1875 Connecticut Avenue, NW, Suite 300
Washington, DC 20009-9110
(202) 332-9110
www.cspinet.org

Centers for Disease Control, Division of Nutrition and Physical Activity
4770 Buford Highway, NE, MS/K-24
Atlanta, GA 30341
(770) 488-5820
www.cdc.gov/nccdphp/dnpa

Food and Nutrition Information Center
National Agricultural Library
10301 Baltimore Avenue, Room 105
Beltsville, MD 20705
(301) 504-5414
fnic.nal.usda.gov

Gatorade Sports Science Institute
617 West Main Street
Barrington, IL 60010
(800) 616-4774
www.gssiweb.com

Institute of Medicine
500 Fifth Street NW
Washington, DC 20001
(202) 334-2352
www.iom.edu

International Food Information Council Foundation
1100 Connecticut Avenue, NW
Suite 430
Washington, DC 20036
(202) 296-6540
www.ific.org

Maternal and Child Health Bureau
Parklawn Building Room 18-05
5600 Fishers Lane
Rockville, Maryland 20857
(301) 443-2170
mchb.hrsa.gov

National Alliance For Youth Sports
2050 Vista Parkway
West Palm Beach, Florida 33411
(561) 684-1141
www.nays.org

National Association of Girls and Women in Sport
1900 Association Dr.
Reston, VA 20191
(703) 476-3400
www.aahperd.org/nagws

National Association of Governor's Councils on Physical Fitness and Sport
65 Niagara Square, Room 607
Buffalo, NY 14022
(716) 583-0521
www.physicalfitness.org/programs.html

National Association of School Nurses
8484 Georgia Avenue, Suite 420
Silver Spring, Maryland 20910
(240) 821-1130
www.nasn.org

National Center for Health Statistics
3311 Toledo Road
Hyattsville, MD 20782
(800) 232-4636
www.cdc.gov/nchs

National Coalition for Promoting Physical Activity
1100 H Street, NW, Suite 510
Washington, D.C. 20005
(202) 454-7521
www.ncppa.org

National Food Service Management Institute
The University of Mississippi
6 Jeanette Phillips Drive
P.O. Drawer 188
University, MS 38677
(800) 321-3054
www.nfsmi.org

National Heart, Lung, and Blood Institute
P.O. Box 30105
Bethesda, MD 20824
(301) 592-8573
www.nhlbi.nih.gov

National Institute for Child Health and Human Development
P.O. Box 3006
Rockville, MD 20847
(800) 370-2943
www.nichd.nih.gov

National Institute of Mental Health
6001 Executive Boulevard, Room 8184, MSC 9663
Bethesda, MD 20892
(866) 615-6464
www.nimh.nih.gov

National Recreation and Parks Association
22377 Belmont Ridge Rd.
Ashburn, VA 20148
(703) 858-0784
www.nrpa.org

National School Board's Association's School Health program
1680 Duke Street
Alexandria, VA 22314
(703) 838-6722
www.nsba.org/schoolhealth

North American Association for the Study of Obesity
8630 Fenton Street, Suite 918
Silver Spring, MD 20910
(301) 563-6526
www.naaso.org

Nutrition.gov
Nutrition.gov Staff
10301 Baltimore Avenue
Beltsville, MD 20705-2351
www.nutrition.gov

Office of Disease Prevention and Health Promotion
Office of Public Health and Science, Office of the Secretary
1101 Wootton Parkway, Suite LL100
Rockville, MD 20852
(240) 453-8280
odphp.osophs.dhhs.gov

PE 4 Life
127 West 10th Street, Suite 101
Kansas City, MO 64105
(816) 472-7345
www.pe4life.org
President's Council on Physical Fitness and Sports

Department W
200 Independence Ave., SW, Room 738-H
Washington, D.C. 20201
202-690-9000
www.fitness.gov

Society for Nutrition Education
7150 Winton Drive, Suite 300
Indianapolis, IN 46268
(800) 235-6690
www.sne.org

Weight-Control Information Network (WIN)
1 WIN Way
Bethesda, MD 20892
(877) 946-4627
www.win.niddk.nih.gov

Women's Sports Foundation
Eisenhower Park
East Meadow, NY 11554
(800) 227-3988
www.womenssportsfoundation.org

INDEX

ABOUT THE AUTHOR

David Campos began his education career more than 15 years ago when he started teaching second grade. He later entered graduate school, taught ESL, and worked in corporate training and development. In 1996, he earned his Ph.D. at The University of Texas at Austin specializing in learning disabilities and behavior disorders. His first job in academia was at Roosevelt University (Chicago, IL) where he was an assistant professor in the College of Education. There he served as Director of the Metropolitan Institute for Teaching and Learning and was an acting assistant dean of academic affairs. After earning rank and tenure he accepted an associate professor of education position at the University of the Incarnate Word (San Antonio, TX).

He has written three books grounded in youth sexuality: *Sex, Youth, and Sex Education*; *Diverse Sexuality in Schools*; and *Understanding Gay and Lesbian Youth*. He also co-authored a resource text and evaluation instrument for teachers of English language learners titled, *Practical Ideas that Really Work for English Language Learners*. His peer-reviewed articles focus on constructivist teaching and authentic assessment by way of African American visionaries. In 2004, he traveled to China as a Fulbright Scholar.

Printed in the United Kingdom
by Lightning Source UK Ltd.
132861UK00001B/112/A